DIY
LOW BACK PAIN RELIEF

9 Ways To Fix Low Back Pain So You Can Feel Like Yourself Again

Morgan Sutherland, L.M.T.

CONTENTS

Medical Disclaimer 4

Introduction 5

Why Should You Trust Me? 7

Way# 1: Sit Right 9

Way #2: Get Up, Stand Up 13

Way #3: Reverse Bad Posture 17

Way #4: Build a Strong Core 26

Way #5: Stretch Your Back 39

Way #6: Pose like a Yogi 51

Way #7: Roll Out the Knots on Your Own 60

Way #8: Sleep This Way 69

Way #9a: Get a Deep Tissue Massage 74

Way #9b: Enhance Your Massage with Cupping 80

Conclusion 85

References 86

About the Author 90

Copyright © 2016 by Morgan Sutherland. All rights reserved.

No part of this book may be reproduced in any form without permission in writing from the author. Reviewers may quote brief passages in reviews. The information contained in this book is current at the time of this writing. Although all attempts have been made to verify the information provided in this publication, neither the author nor the publisher assumes any responsibility for errors, omissions, or contrary interpretations of the subject matter herein.

This book is for entertainment purposes only. The views expressed are those of the author alone and should not be taken as expert instruction or commands. The reader is responsible for his or her own actions.

At times links might be used to illustrate a point, technique, or best practice. These will reference products I have found useful, but please do your own research, make appropriate comparisons, and form your own decisions as to which product will work best for you. Even though it is an accepted industry practice, I have not used any affiliate links, in order to avoid any possible conflicts of interest. Links to my own website or products are used to illustrate points, because they are the examples with which I am most familiar.

Medical Disclaimer

The information provided in this book is not intended to be a substitute for professional medical advice, diagnosis or treatment. Never disregard or delay seeking professional medical advice, because of something you read in this book. Never rely on information in this book in place of seeking professional medical advice.

Morgan Sutherland is not responsible or liable for any advice, course of treatment, diagnosis, other information, services and/or products that you obtain in this book. You are encouraged to consult with your doctor or healthcare provider with regard to the information contained in this book. After reading this book, you are encouraged to review the information carefully with your professional healthcare provider.

Personal Disclaimer

I am not a doctor. The information I provide is based on my personal experiences and research as a licensed massage therapist. Any recommendations I make about posture, exercise, stretching and massage should be discussed between you and your professional healthcare provider to prevent any risk to your health.

Introduction

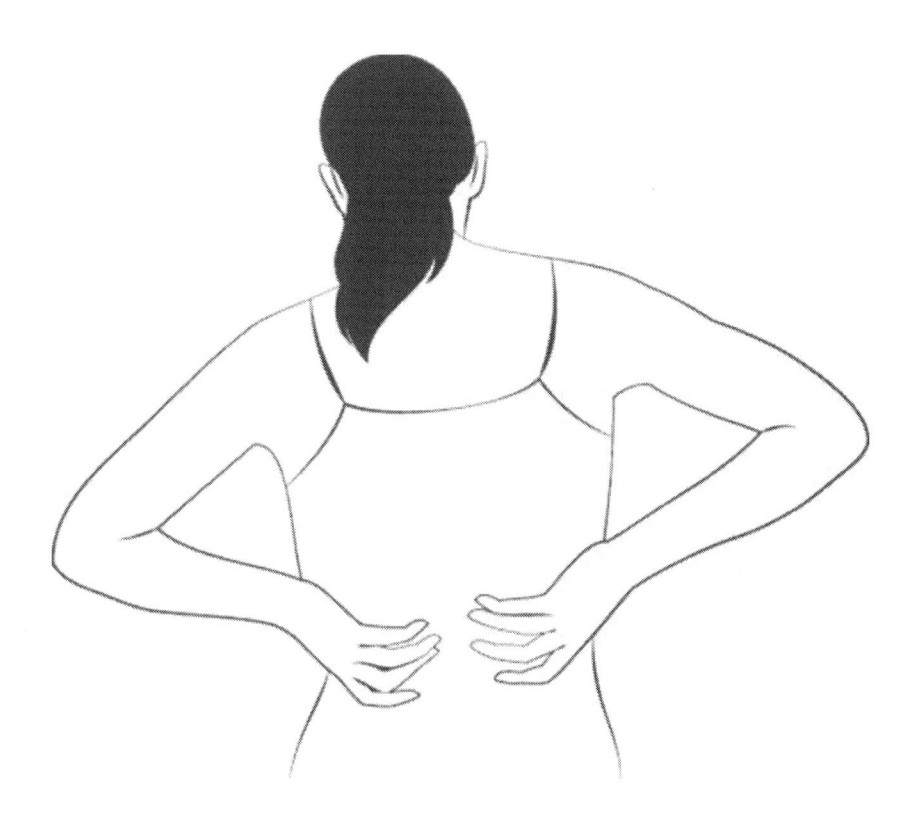

Got Back Pain? Now What?

Chronic pain, affecting approximately 100 million people each year, is classified as pain persisting for 30 to 60 days or more. Low back pain is the most common kind of chronic pain complaint. When the body's pain signals keep firing in the nervous system for this length of time, it can have draining effect on a person's quality of life—physically, mentally and spiritually.

In the United States, 8 out of 10 people will experience low back pain at sometime in their lives. Low back pain is the second most frequent reason for doctor visits, next to the common cold, and it is the leading cause of job-related disabilities.

When sudden and acute back pain strikes, it can cause intense shooting or stabbing pain that dramatically limits movement. This is often to the point that standing upright can feel like a Sisyphean task—repeatedly rolling the same rock up the hill without any relief. This pain can last anywhere from a few days to weeks.

Acute back pain is generally the result of a strained muscle, that's when the muscle or tendon is ripped or torn, from overstretching it, or by pulling the muscle in one direction while it is contracting in the other direction. Muscle strains are typically caused from a fall, careless lifting technique, poor posture or a sudden movement.

Finding a quick fix for back pain relief can lead down a dark path of taking painkillers. This will temporarily mask the pain, but can pack a stealthy punch of potentially dangerous side effects.

In some cases, going the bed-rest route and taking a day or two off from work to "rest your back" can quickly resolve a temporary back strain. However, prolonged immobilization might have adverse effects, such as depression, blood clots in the legs, muscle atrophy or even muscle splinting (that's when the muscle becomes extremely tight and contracted).

In fact, a 1995 Finnish study found that people, following the onset of low back pain, who kept moving without bed rest had better back flexibility than those who rested in bed for a week.

In the following pages, you will learn how reversing bad posture, building a strong core and incorporating a regular stretching and massage routine are essential steps in maintaining a pain-free back and feeling like yourself again.

Why Should You Trust Me?

As a 16-year veteran massage therapist, I've helped thousands of clients suffering with chronic pain and sports injuries with a combination of deep tissue massage and cupping. For the past three consecutive years, I've been awarded the Angie's List Super Service Award, an honor given annually to approximately 5 percent of all the companies rated on Angie's List, the nation's leading provider of consumer reviews about local service companies.

The majority of my clients seek me out for help with relief of chronic and acute back pain. For some, a 60- or 90-minute massage is enough to make them magically float off my table feeling rejuvenated and pain-free. However, countless clients crave advice about what they can do outside the treatment room to manage their pain. I wanted to provide them with a sequence of stretches, strengthening exercises and self-massage methods that would give them control over their pain, and that's where the idea for this book materialized.

How Did I Get into Massage?

After college, motivated to make a difference in the world, I decided to volunteer and teach English in Costa Rica. On returning home, I continued teaching English at a prominent language school, but realized that I had lost my passion for the profession.

Deciding to become a massage therapist was deeply influenced by growing up with a filmmaker father whose life was inundated with pain patches, neck braces and high stress. The countless hours perched behind his editors like a crazed puppeteer, took an inevitable toll on his body and well-being.

DIY Low Back Pain Relief

For as long as I can remember, my father had a standing weekly massage appointment to manage his aches and pains. He would return noticeably more relaxed and less cranky.

Seeing how my father benefited from regular massage, I decided to book a session with his massage therapist in efforts to explore the idea of changing careers and becoming a massage therapist. The massage experience made such a positive impact on me that I quickly enrolled in massage therapy school and soon after realized my true calling.

Way# 1: Sit Right

In today's culture, everyone's constantly plugged into some device, be it a computer, laptop, tablet or smart phone. Sedentary lifestyles inevitably result in clocking thousands of hours with our bodies resembling a human question mark—our heads jutting forward, our shoulders rounding and our stomachs getting closer to our knees.

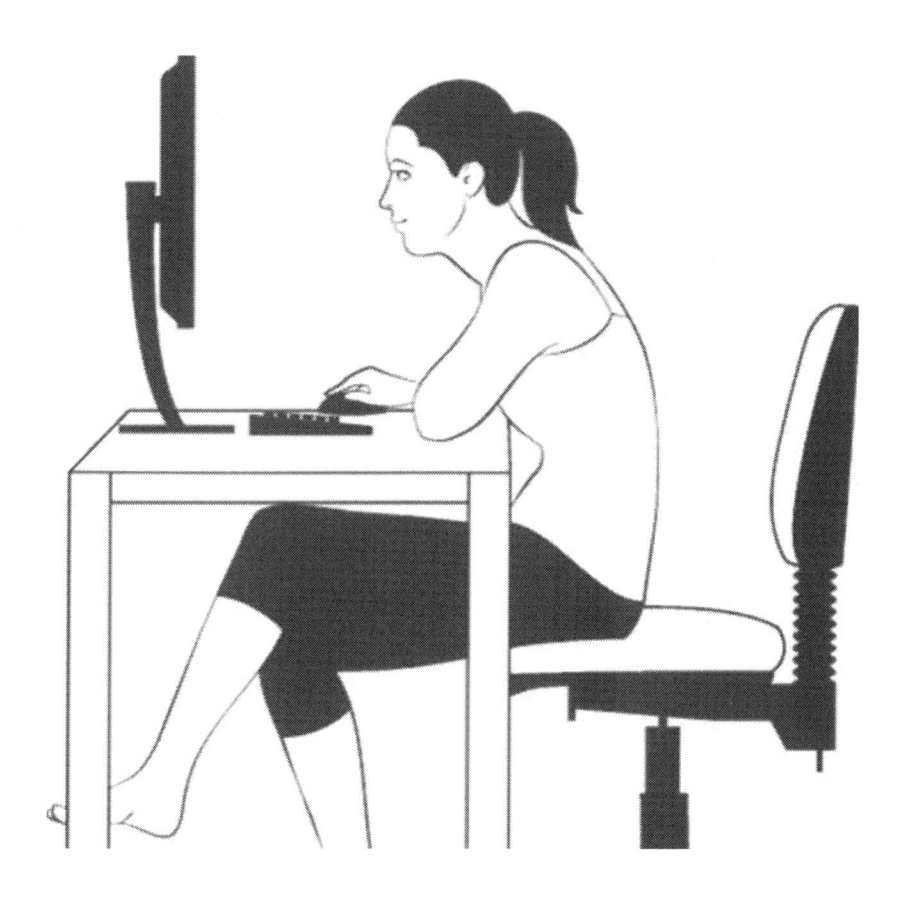

Prolonged Sitting and Back Pain

Sitting for too long causes your low back muscles and hip flexors (the muscles that allow you to lift your knees and bend at your waist) to become short and tight. Slumped over in a chair all day also makes your abdominal muscles slowly lose tone and your glutes (also known at the buttocks) to become overstretched and weak.

Another phenomenon that happens with prolonged sitting is that it causes an anterior (or front) tilt, which is an adaptive shortening of the hip flexor muscles. When moving from a prolonged sitting position to an upright one, the shortened hip flexors inevitably pull on the muscle attachments of the lumbar (low back) spine causing an anterior shift in the hips. This can put unwanted strain on the low back, exaggerate the lumbar curve and potentially cause a bulging or herniated disc.

Sit the Right Way

If you have to sit for extended periods of time, maintaining good posture is key! Chronic slouching or leaning to one side, even if these positions make the pain subside, are bad habits that propagate back pain.

The National Institute of Neurological Disorders and Stroke recommends sitting in a chair with good low back support. If sitting for a long time, you should rest your feet on a low stool. If possible, switch sitting positions and get up and walk around a bit throughout the day.

Reprogram Your Body to Sit Correctly in Eight Moves

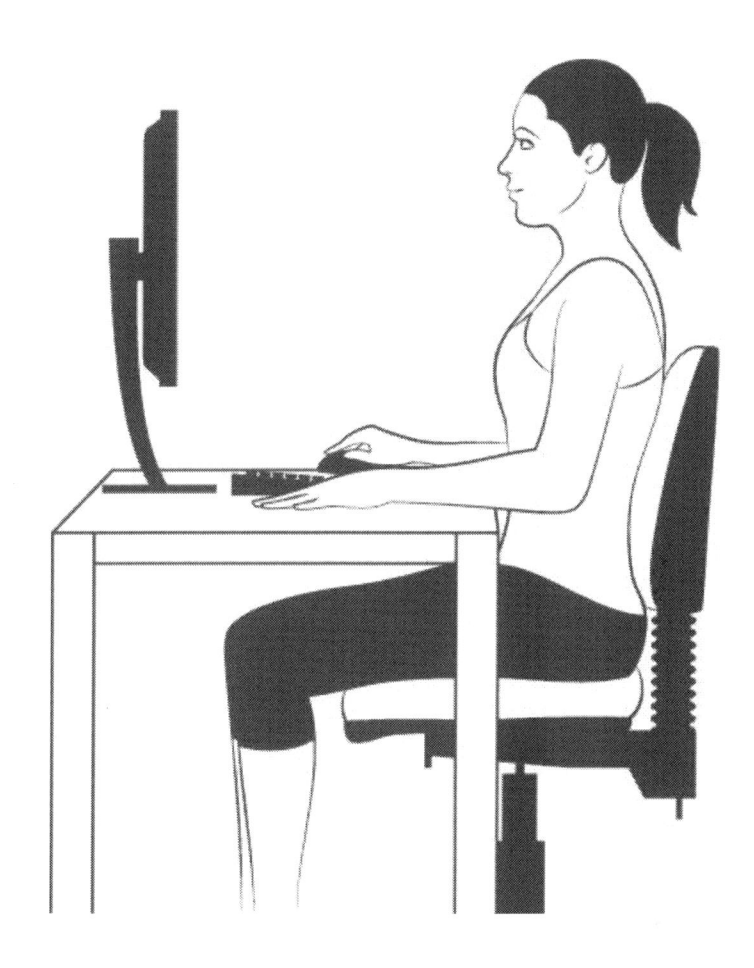

1. Sit back in your chair. If you can't sit back, support your low back with a lumbar roll, rolled towel or small pillow.

2. Don't lean forward and sit on the edge of your chair. This will cause your low back to arch, your head to drop forward and your shoulders to round.

3. Drop your shoulders and keep them relaxed, so it doesn't look like you're wearing them as earrings.

4. Keep your arms close to your sides.

5. Make sure your elbows are bent 90 degrees.

6. Stretch the top of your head toward the ceiling, and tuck your chin in slightly.

7. Keep your upper back and neck comfortably straight by rolling your shoulders back and tucking in your tummy about 20 percent.

8. Place your feet flat on the floor, pointing them forward so your knees are level with your hips. If necessary, prop up your feet with a footstool or other support.

Way #2: Get Up, Stand Up

Sometimes you can't avoid stooping. When you are gardening or doing household chores that require you to bend over, make sure to keep your knees bent and your back straight.

Lifting objects with a rounded back can put unwanted pressure on the vertebral discs (bones in the spinal column) and potentially injure your low back. Keeping the body upright, maintaining a natural lumbar curve is a better option when lifting.

According to the American Academy of Orthopaedic Surgeons, if you are going to lift something:

- Position yourself as close to the object as possible, so that you are more stable.

- Keep your feet shoulder width apart to create a solid base of support.

- Always bend at the knees, tighten your abdominals and lift with your legs.

When you stand for long periods of time, your lumbar curve can become excessive, and pain can result (this is called lordosis). The illustration below is a perfect example of a person with poor standing posture. You've probably seen someone like this before, waiting to place her order at your favorite coffee shop, with her head stooped over her phone like the hunchback Quasimodo.

DIY Low Back Pain Relief

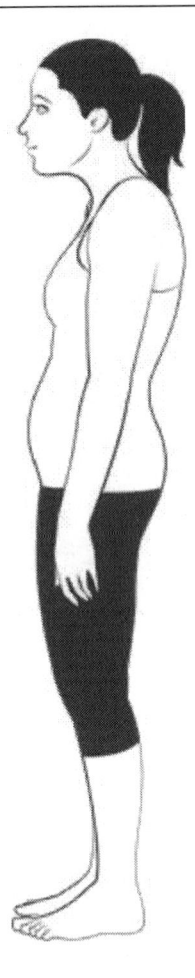

You'll notice the shoulders are rounded, causing the upper back muscles to overstretch and tighten up the chest muscles. This posture can potentially compress the brachial plexus, which is the network of nerves that originate in the neck and feed into the armpit region and down into the arms. A brachial plexus impingement can lead to a number of problems from numbness in the hands, to thoracic outlet syndrome or carpal tunnel-like symptoms. In this hunched posture, the abdominals are loose, which gives them an exaggerated lumbar curve.

Way #3: Reverse Bad Posture

This kind of slouched posture can trigger low back pain, neck pain, headaches, tendonitis and also lead to worn-out, imbalanced muscles. It's like an energy vampire, sucking away any vibrant spirit you possess. I'm going to show you how to combat this slouched posture in six moves.

How to Stand the Right Way in Six Moves

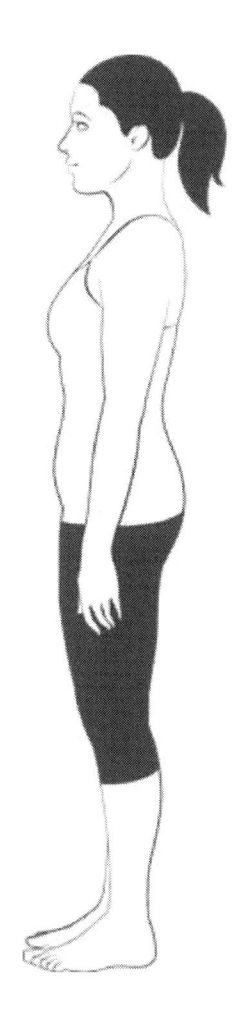

Good posture allows your spine to be aligned and balanced. You can breathe deeply because your lungs and diaphragm have more space to expand and contract. Not only will you feel more energized and less worn down, but you'll also look good and be twice as likely to smile.

1. First, stand up with your feet pointing forward or slightly turned inward.

2. Now, squeeze your glutes tightly and rotate your feet inward, so that your big toes slightly turn toward each other.

3. Tighten your thighs, about 50 percent.

4. Slightly tighten your abdominals, only about 20 percent.

5. Now, roll your shoulders back. This brings your shoulder blades closer together and your chest moves up and forward.

6. Last, turn your hands so that your thumbs are facing forward.

Voila! Your now have perfect standing posture.

Way #3: Reverse Bad Posture

Neglected postures, such as rounding your low back while sitting for extended periods of time in front of the computer, standing for hours stooped over, sleeping improperly and lifting poorly, can all lead to chronic back pain.

Maintaining the natural lumbar curve in your low back is essential to preventing posture-related back pain. This natural curve works as a shock absorber, helping to distribute weight along the length of your spine.

Adjusting postural distortions can help stop back pain. A basic remedy to sitting all day is to simply get up! Frequently getting up from a seated position and doing specific, quick and easy realignment exercises can help you reeducate your muscles from getting stuck in a concaved Cro-Magnon posture.

Six Exercises to Reverse Bad Posture

1. Chin Tuck

Did you know that for every inch the head moves forward in posture, its weight on your neck and upper back muscles increases by 10 pounds? For example, a human head weighing 12 pounds held forward only 3 inches from the shoulders, results in 42 pounds of pressure on the neck and upper back muscles.

The Chin Tuck exercise can help reverse forward-head posture by strengthening the neck muscles.

DIY Low Back Pain Relief

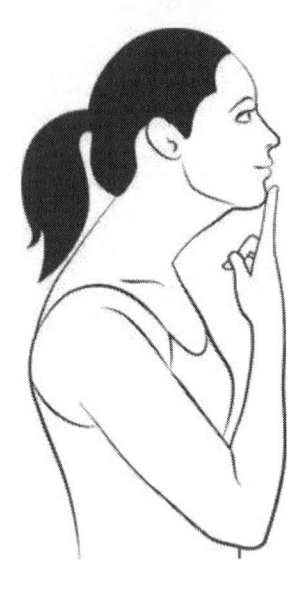

This exercise can be done sitting or standing. Start with your shoulders rolled back and down. While looking straight ahead, place two fingers on your chin, slightly tuck your chin and move your head back. Hold for 3 to 5 seconds and then release. Repeat 10 times.

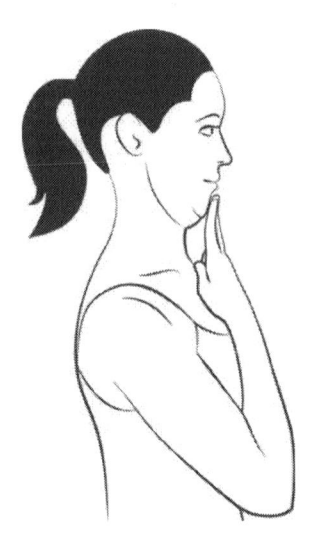

Tip: The more of a double chin you create the better the results. If you're in a parked car, try doing the Chin Tuck pressing the back of your head into the headrest for 3 to 5 seconds. Do 15 to 20 repetitions.

2. Wall Angel

Keep your feet about 4 inches away from the wall and maintain a slight bend in your knees. Your glutes, spine and head should all be against the wall as you bring the shoulder blades together and squeeze, forming the letter "W" with your arms. Hold for 3 seconds.

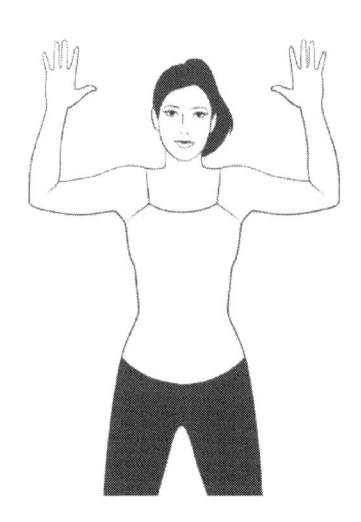

Now raise your arms up to form the letter "Y." Make sure not to shrug your shoulders to your ears. Repeat this 10 times, starting at "W," holding for 3 seconds and then raising your arms into a "Y." Do two to three sets.

DIY Low Back Pain Relief

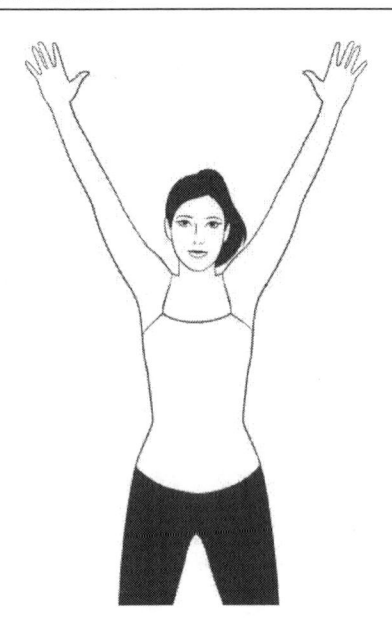

3. Doorway Stretch—The Contract-Relax-Stretch Version

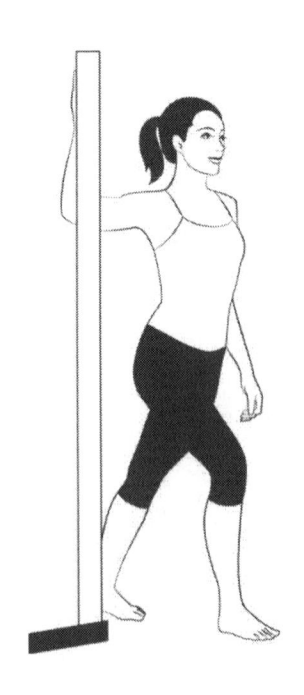

Way #3: Reverse Bad Posture

This exercise loosens those tight chest muscles.

First, reach your arm outward 90 degrees. Then, place your hand on the doorjamb and lean forward.

Slowly, lean into your raised arm and push against the doorjamb for 7 to 10 seconds. Relax and then stretch your bent arm back and stretch your chest for 7 to 10 seconds. Repeat this stretch two to three times.

4. Hip Flexor Stretch

To effectively stretch the hip flexors, first kneel on your right knee, with toes down, and place your left foot flat on the floor in front of you.

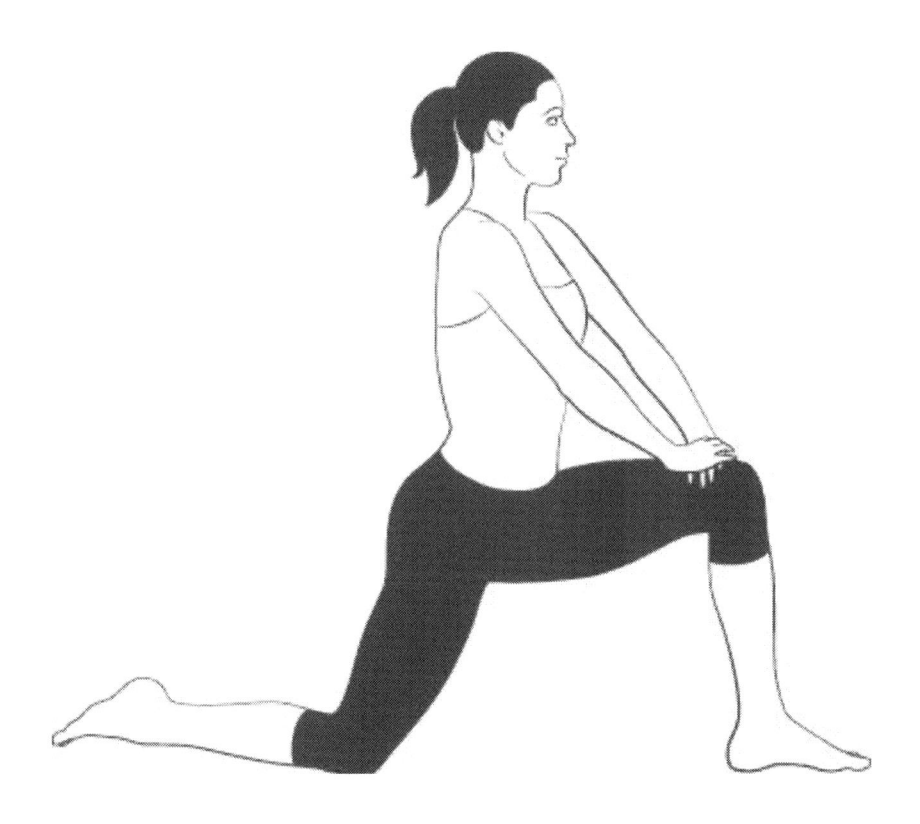

DIY Low Back Pain Relief

Place both hands on your left thigh and press your hips forward until you feel a good stretch in the hip flexors.

Contract your abdominals and slightly tilt your pelvis back while keeping your chin parallel to the floor. Hold this pose for 20 to 30 seconds, and then switch sides.

Tip: To accentuate this stretch, reach your hands over your head and arch your body back.

Way #3: Reverse Bad Posture

The Following Two Exercises Require a Resistance Band[1]

5. The X-Move (also called Seated Row)

This exercise helps strengthen your upper back muscles, especially the ones between your shoulder blades, called the rhomboids.

To do the X-Move, sit on the floor with your legs extended forward. Securely wrap the middle of the band around your feet to prevent it from slipping.

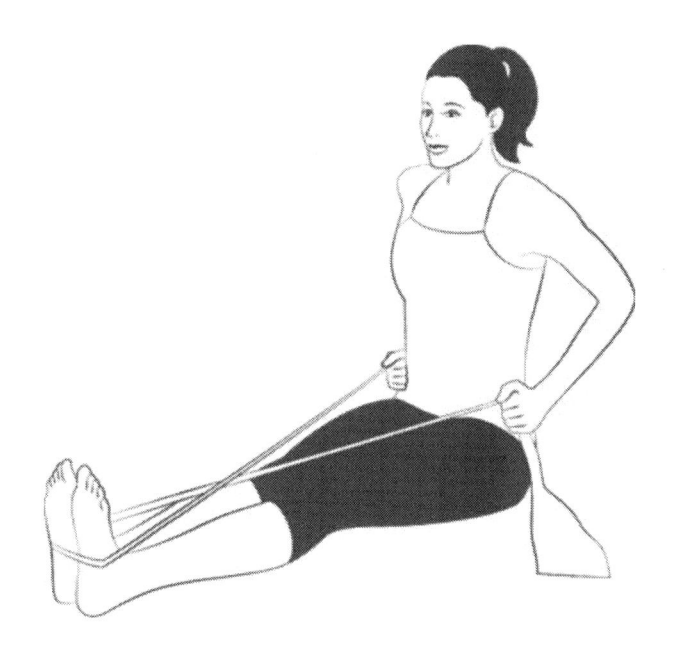

Grasp the ends of the band with your arms extended in front of you so that you form an "X."

---

[1] Sometimes called elastic stretch bands, these are available at fitness centers, athletic stores, department stores, or online.

Pull the ends of the band toward your hips, bending your elbows. Hold and slowly return. Do 8 to 12 repetitions for three sets.

Tip: Keep your knees and back straight.

6. The V-Move (with resistance band[2])

According to a 2013 study by the Scandinavian Society of Clinical Physiology and Nuclear Medicine, 50 percent of office workers will suffer from neck and shoulder pain every year from prolonged periods of poor posture while at work.

According to the researchers, performing this simple resistance-band exercise 2 minutes a day, five times a week, will significantly decrease your neck and shoulder pain and improve your posture.

---

[2] This exercise works better with resistance tubing with handles, but the resistance bands will also work.

Way #3: Reverse Bad Posture

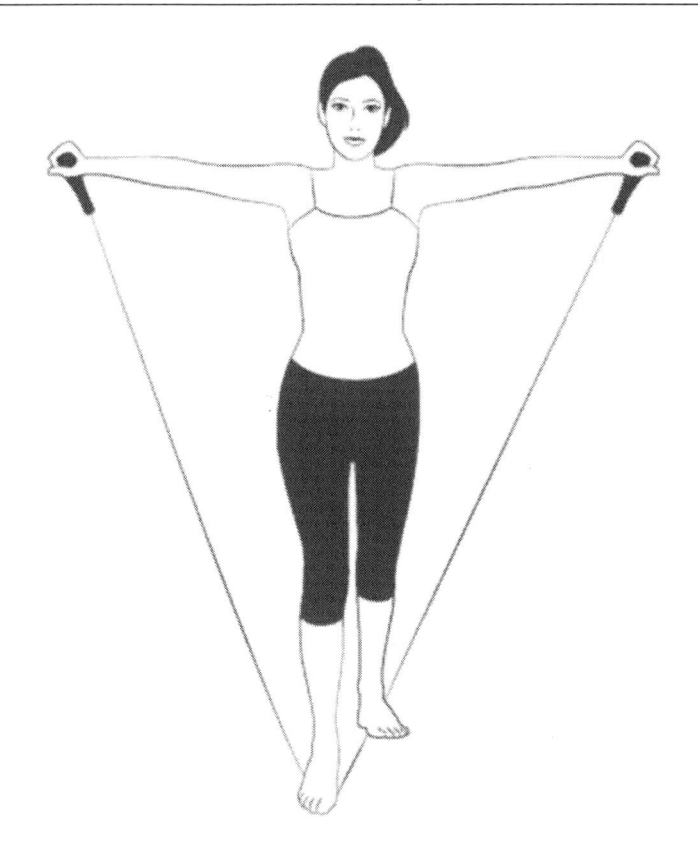

How to Do the Exercise

Assume a staggered stance position. Grasp the handles, or the ends, of the resistance band and lift your arms upward and slightly outward away from your body about 30 degrees.

Keep your elbows bent about 5 degrees. Stop at shoulder level; hold and return.

Make sure to keep your shoulder blades down and avoid shrugging your shoulders and keep your back straight. Repeat this exercise for 2 minutes each day for five (work) days.

Good work!

Way #4: Build a Strong Core

Sedentary lifestyles usually go hand in hand with being unfit and overweight. According to a study published in the *American Journal of Epidemiology*, obese people have a higher prevalence of low back pain than non-overweight individuals.

Another study, published in the *Arthritis & Rheumatology* journal, reported that overweight and obese adults are more likely to have disc degeneration in their low back than normal-weight adults. An excessive anterior tilt in the pelvis coupled with weak abdominal muscles creates an excessive amount of tension in a person's low back. This leads to back pain and the increased likelihood of disc deterioration.

So, it's no secret. If your back is sore and achy, you need to strengthen your core, the abdominal and pelvic muscles that encircle and support the spine.

The "core" consists of specific muscles, which stabilize the spine and pelvis, and run the entire length of the torso. The core muscles make it possible to stand upright, shift your body weight, transfer your energy and move in any direction.

Way #4: Build a Strong Core

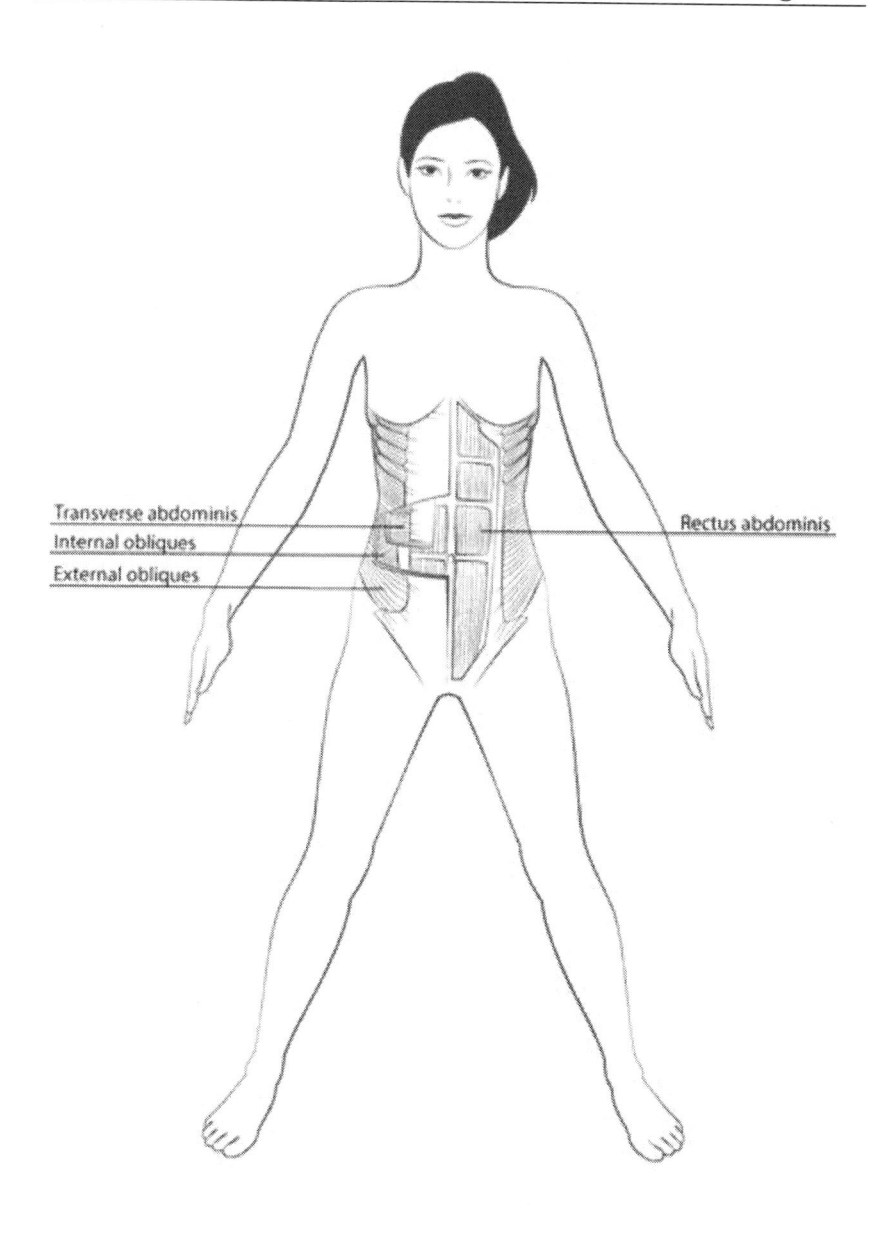

There are four major core muscles: the rectus abdominus, external and internal obliques and the transverse obliques.

The rectus abdominus extends along the front of the abdomen and forms the "six-pack" muscles.

The external obliques are on the side and front of the abdomen, around your waist.

Underneath the external obliques are the internal obliques. Underneath the internal obliques is the transverse abdominus, which wraps around your spine for protection and stability.

Muscles function with an agonist/antagonist response, so if one muscle takes the brunt of the work, the neglected muscle becomes weakened. Weak core muscles diminish a person's natural lumbar curve creating a scenario for crippling back pain. A strong, balanced core helps maintain appropriate posture and reduces strain on the spine.

Way #4: Build a Strong Core

Eight Exercises That Will Strengthen Your Core and Save Your Back!

1. The Plank

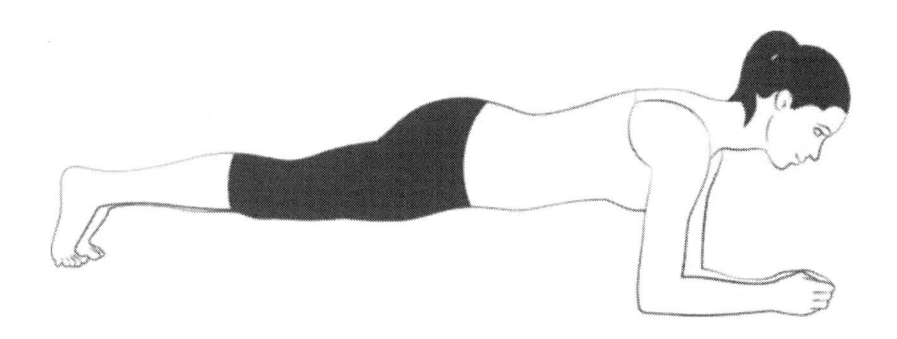

Get into a plank position on the floor with feet hip-width apart and elbows directly under your shoulders.

Brace your core by contracting your abs and attempt to bring your belly button toward your spine.

Keep your back straight and legs and glutes engaged the entire time. Hold this pose for 1 minute.

DIY Low Back Pain Relief

2. The Side Plank

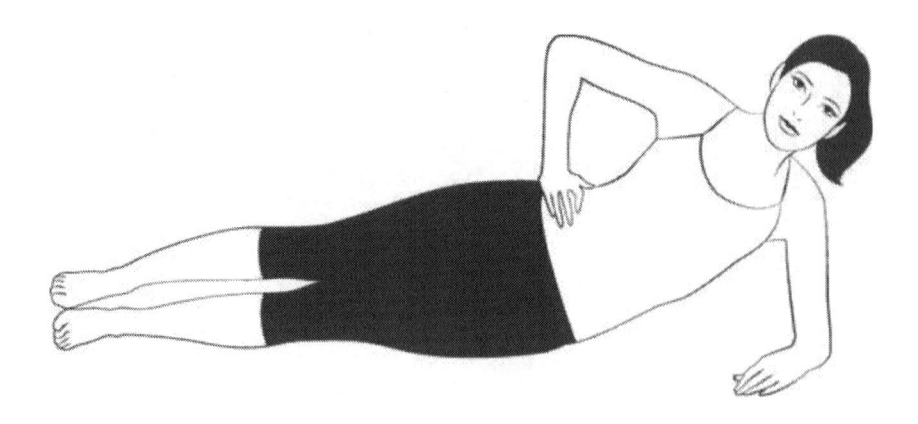

When performing the side plank, start by lying on your side with your forearm on the floor under your shoulder, to prop you up, and then stack your feet on top of each other.

Contract your abdominals and press your forearm into the floor to raise your hips so that your body is straight from your ankles to your shoulders.

Hold this position for 30 to 60 seconds, and then repeat on the other side.

3. Single-Leg Lowering

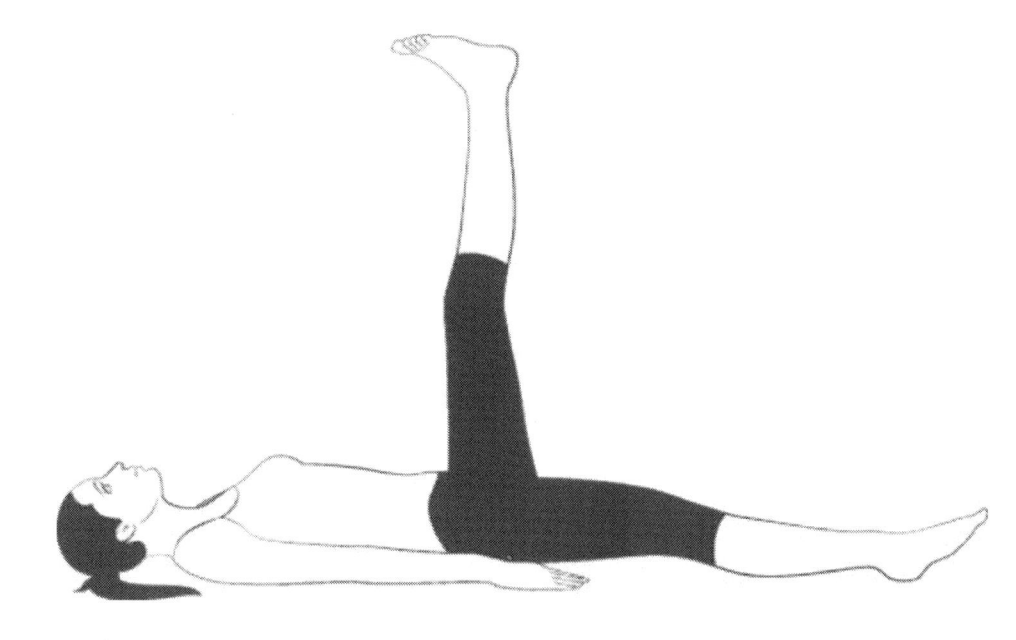

Begin this exercise by lying on your back with both legs extended straight up.

Keeping your legs straight, slowly lower your left leg until it's a few inches off the floor (make sure to lead with your heel, keeping your foot flexed).

Return to the starting position, and then repeat this exercise with your right leg. That's one repetition. Do this 8 to 12 times on both sides.

4. The Pilates' Hundreds

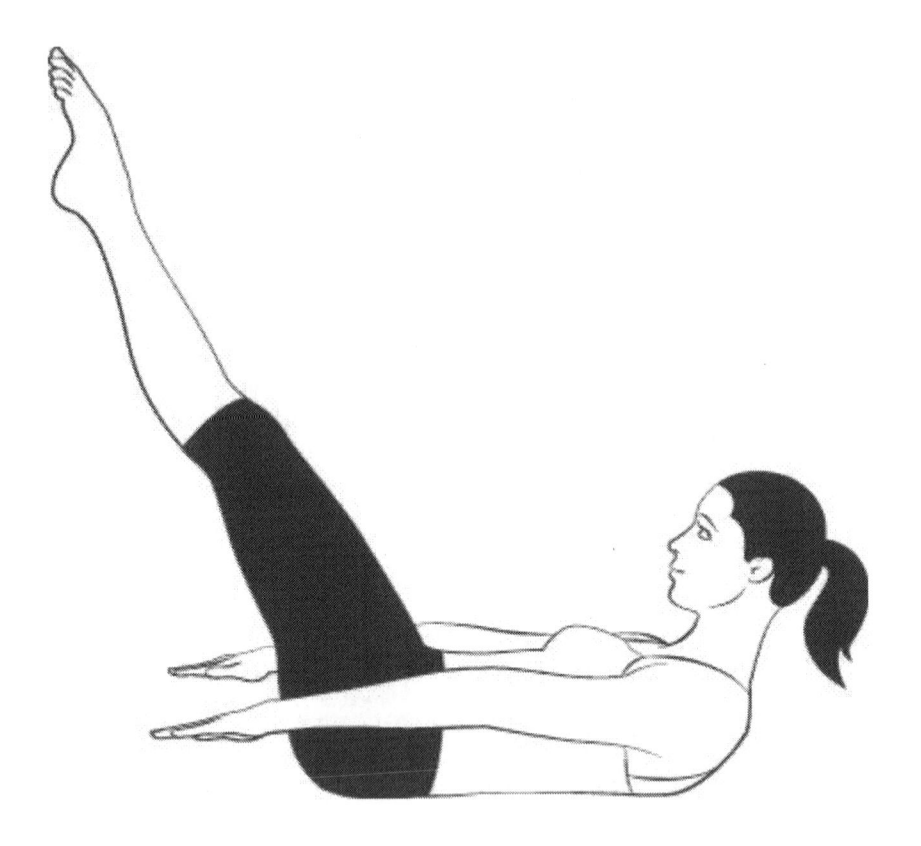

Begin by lying on your back, keeping the small of your back pressed down toward the floor, your abs tight, legs extended and arms at your sides.

Lift your legs straight up and then lower them to a 45-degree angle.

Inhale deeply, and as you exhale, lift through your shoulder blades and extend your arms forward, keeping them parallel to the floor.

Way #4: Build a Strong Core

Now, quickly pulse your arms up and down as you inhale for a count of five and exhale for a count of five.

Do this for 1 minute and then slowly lower your shoulders, and pull your knees to your chest to stretch.

5. Superman (or Superwoman) Exercises

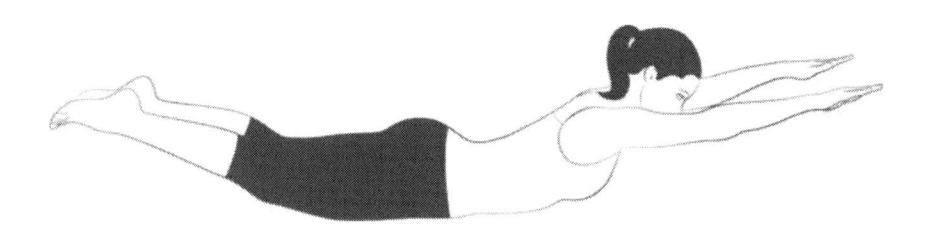

Lie face down on the floor on your stomach with arms and legs extended and your neck in a neutral position.

Keeping your arms and legs straight and your torso stationary, simultaneously lift your arms and legs up toward the ceiling to form an elongated "U" shape with your body—back arched and arms and legs lifted several inches off the floor.

Hold for 2 to 5 seconds and then lower your arms and legs to complete one. Do 3 sets of 12.

6. The Old-Fashioned Push-Up

Not just a chest builder, the push-up also works your core. If you are unable to push up with your legs fully extended, place your knees on the floor to begin with.

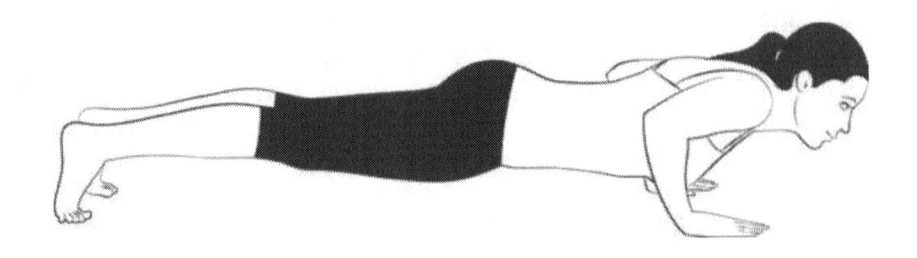

Start on the floor and bring yourself into the push-up position with your hands placed directly under your shoulders and your palms on the floor, your back flat and your toes curled on the floor (or knees on the floor).

Slowly lower yourself by bending your elbows and bringing them out to the side until you are hovering just above the floor.

Make sure you keep your back flat and your abs pulled in (toward your spine).

Way #4: Build a Strong Core

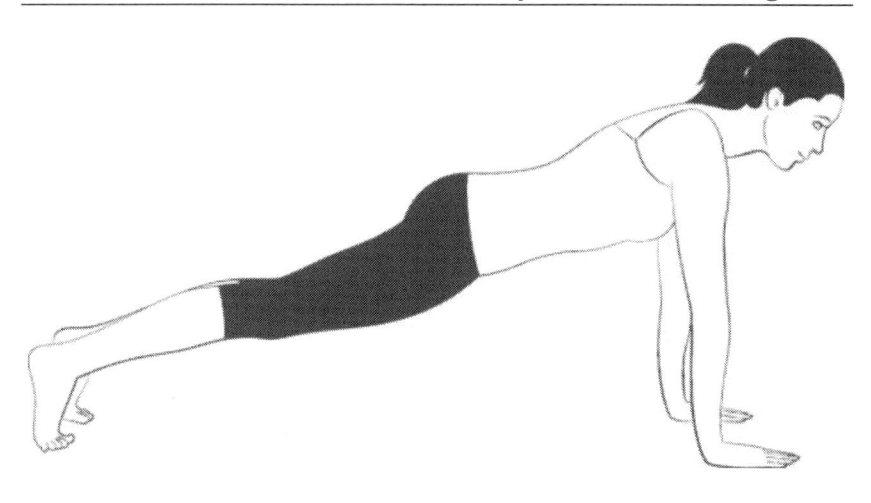

Next, extend your arms and return to your starting position. Try to do 10 to 20 repetitions, or as many as you can, using good form.

7. Bridge with Knee Squeeze

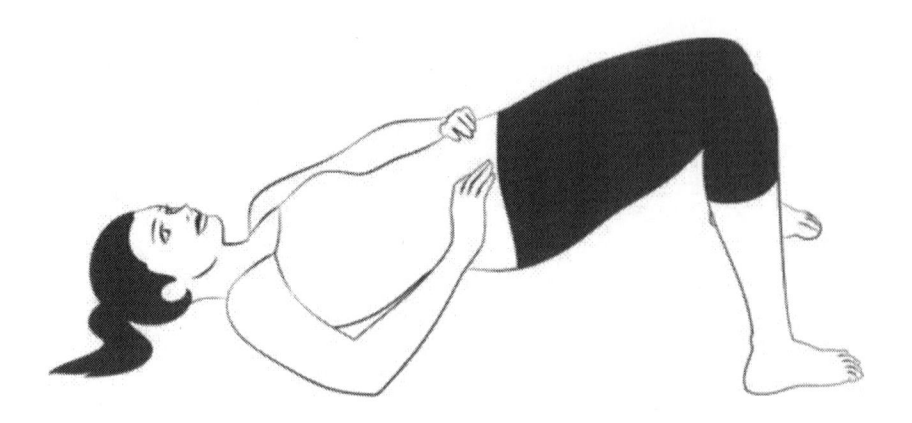

For this bridge move, begin by lying on the floor and simultaneously lifting your hips and squeezing your glutes together. Hold for 2 to 3 seconds and then relax. Do 10 to 15 repetitions.

Next, raise the hips and squeeze your knees together. Hold for 2 to 3 seconds and then relax. Do 10 to 15 repetitions.

Take it to the next level by slightly lifting one foot off the floor. Make sure to keep your hips parallel to the floor.

Way #4: Build a Strong Core

8. Hamstring Curl Bridge

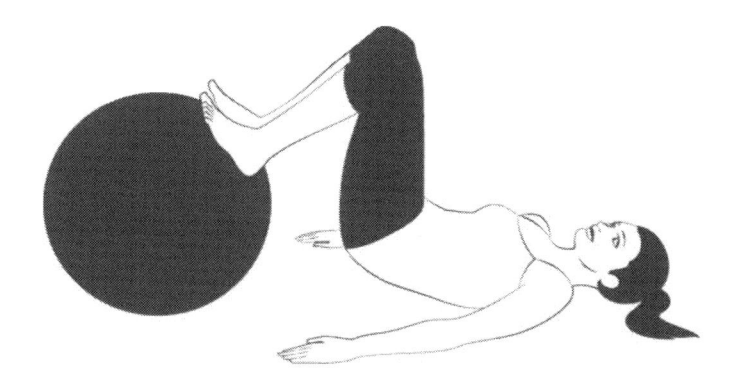

This second bridge move involves placing your feet on a gymnastic ball[3] and slowly lifting your hips.

As you lift, roll the ball away from your body and then back toward your body. That's one repetition.

Repeat this move 10 to 15 times, doing your best to keep your the hips lifted the entire time.

You're feeling the burn, right? You did amazing!

Bonus Move: Resistance Band Hip-Strengthening Technique

Hip abductor weakness has been implicated as a factor in chronic low back pain. A painful or weak gluteus medius muscle (that's the muscle in the hip that allows you to laterally rotate the hip) will force a person to lean toward the involved side to place the center of gravity over the hip. This can ultimately lead to abnormal loading of the lumbar spine and subsequent low back pain.

---

[3] Also called a gym ball, exercise ball, or fitness ball, you can purchase this item at a fitness center, athletic store, department store, or online.

DIY Low Back Pain Relief

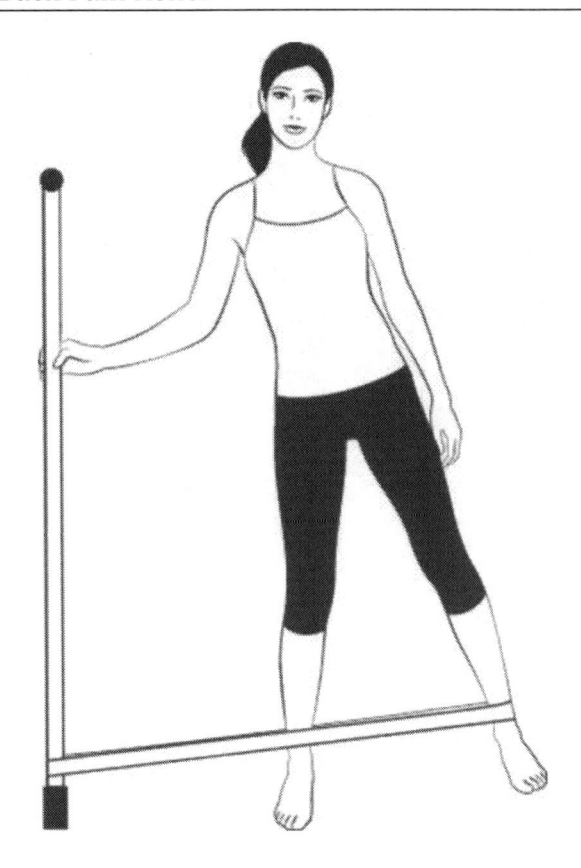

Do three sets of 8 to 12 repetitions.

Now you have an arsenal of moves to build a strong core and stop back pain in its tracks.[4]

---

[4] Using an elastic loop band instead of a regular resistance band might make this hip abduction exercise easier.

Way #5: Stretch Your Back

If your low back is feeling stiff, achy and about to spasm (or you're already there), then do the following nine stretches. Try performing this sequence three times a day. Once the pain is considerably less, you can reduce the sequence to once a day and ultimately three to four times per week.

When you're ready to start, lie down on the bed or floor (preferably on a carpet, rug or yoga mat).

Pelvic Tilt Warmup

Lie on your back with your knees bent and feet flat on the floor. In this relaxed position, the small of your back will not be touching the floor.

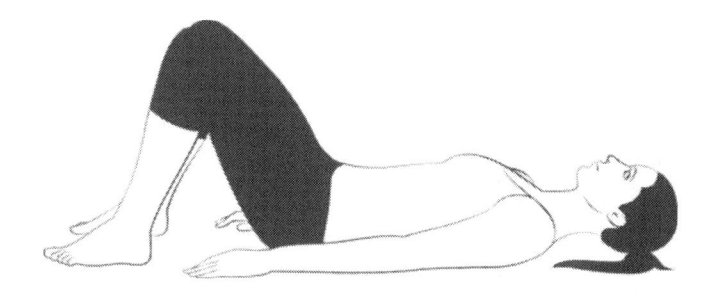

Perform a pelvic tilt by tightening your abdominal muscles so that the small of your back presses against the floor. Hold for 5 seconds, and then relax. Repeat this move three times and gradually build to 10 repetitions.

Next, take a deep breath and on the exhale contract your abdominals, pulling your belly button towards your spine. Hold for 5 to 10 seconds. Repeat 10 times.

Now, you are ready to begin stretching.

Nine Stretching Sequences for Chronic Back Pain

1. Hamstring Floor Stretch

Desk jockeys who sit all day long are guaranteed to have tight hamstrings. These are the group of muscles that help bend your knee and extend your hips. They are located on the back of your upper thigh.

When the hamstrings are too tight, they can pull the backside of the pelvis downward. This downward pull of the pelvis can cause a flattening of your back, which increases pressure on the bones of your lumbar spine.

If this pulling happens for an extended time period, it causes the muscles in the low back, which hold your body upright, to become weak and start to fatigue as they try to hold your body upright against gravity. For this reason, stretching the hamstrings is crucial to help reduce the strain on your low back.

Way #5: Stretch Your Back

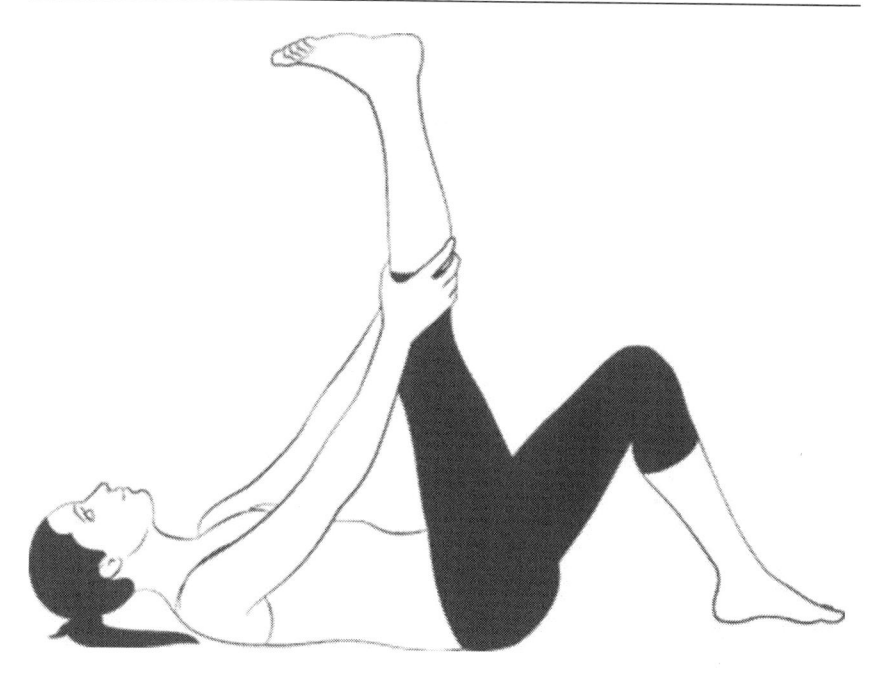

Begin by laying flat on the floor with your knees bent. Contract your abdominals while bringing one leg up, keeping your knee straight. Grasp behind the calf muscle and hold for 30 seconds. Do this two times for each leg.

2. Knees to Chest Stretch

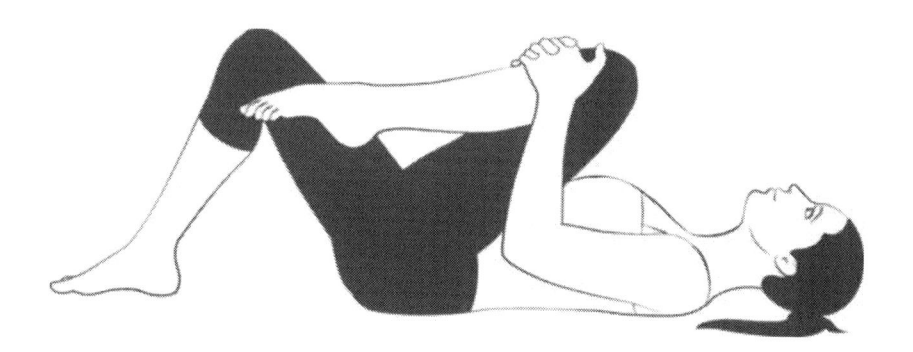

DIY Low Back Pain Relief

While you're still on your back, with your knees bent, grasp your left knee and pull it to your chest. Hold for 20 seconds. With your abdominals contracted, try to straighten your right leg. If you experience any discomfort in your back, leave your right leg bent. Repeat this move with the other leg.

Way #5: Stretch Your Back

3. Spinal Stretch

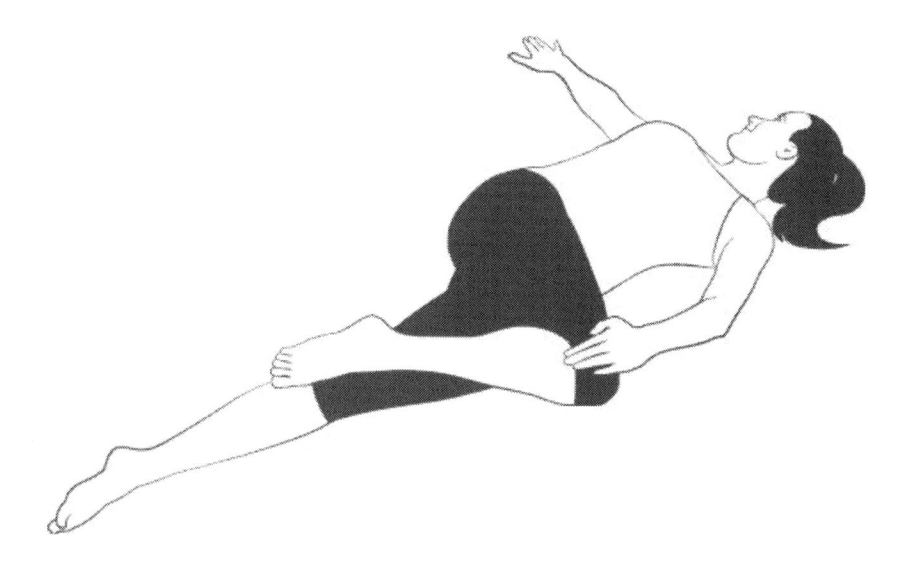

Remain on the floor and stretch both legs out. With your right arm stretched to the right, lift your right knee across your left knee. Contract your abdominals before bringing your knee up and over the leg. Hold for 20 seconds. Repeat this move with the other knee.

4. Seated Hip Stretch

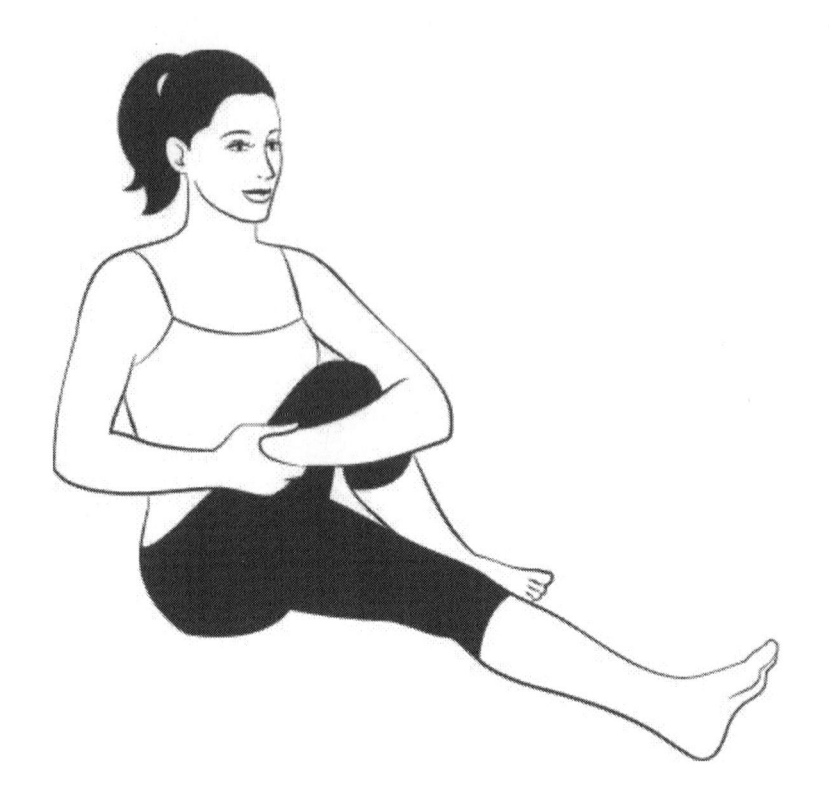

While in a sitting position, cross your right leg over your straightened left leg. Hug your right knee with your left arm, making sure to keep your back straight.

Hold this stretch for 30 to 60 seconds, and then repeat on the opposite side.

5. Piriformis Stretch

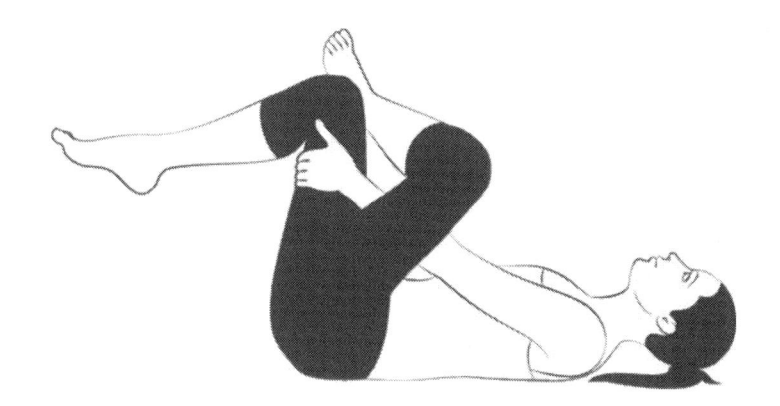

The piriformis is a tiny, pear-shaped muscle deep in the glutes that helps laterally rotate the hip. If gets too tight, it can impinge the sciatica nerve that runs through or under it, causing tremendous pain, tingling and numbness through the glutes and into the lower leg. This condition is called piriformis syndrome.

When performing the piriformis stretch, make sure to contract your abdominals before crossing your leg and resting your foot on the other knee. Hold this stretch for 30 seconds and then repeat with your other leg.

6. Adductor Stretches

The inner thigh muscles, known as the adductors, play a crucial role in movement and stabilization of the legs and pelvis. The adductors help support the pelvis and allow you to bring your legs toward and across the midline of your body. Tight adductors can distort the posture and accentuate the anterior tilt, which contributes to low back pain. Weak adductors can throw off a person's gait and force the body to compensate so as to maintain pelvic stability.

6a. Butterfly Stretch

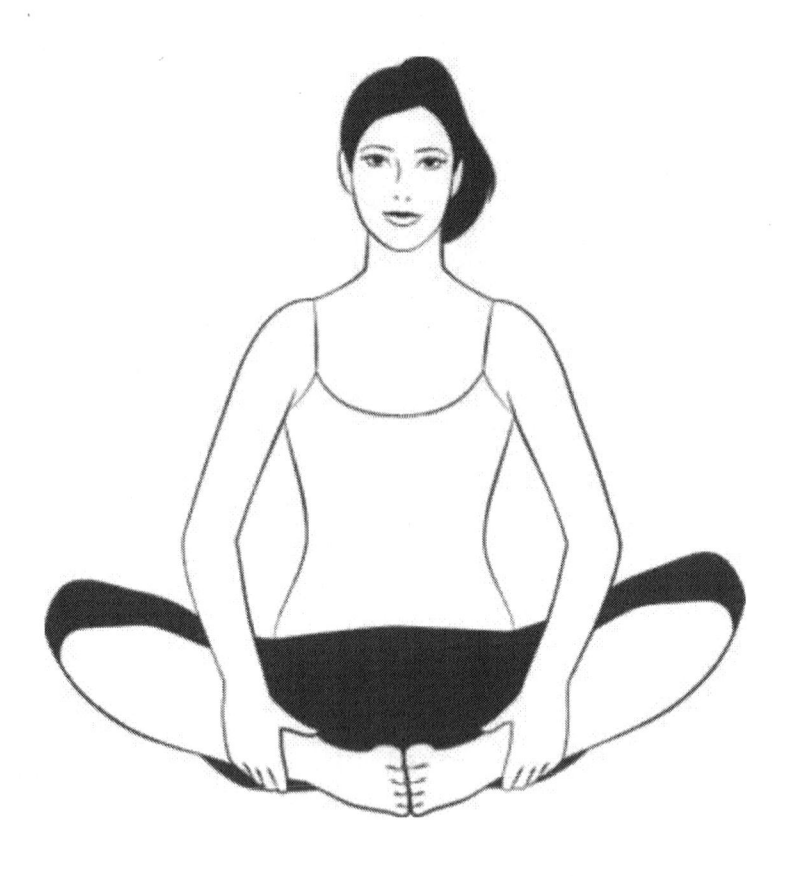

The butterfly stretch is a static stretch that helps to improve the flexibility of your adductors.

First sit on the floor or a mat, open your hips, flex your knees and move your feet together. Grasp your ankles and gently pull them up as you simultaneously push your elbows into your knees. Hold for 30 seconds.

6b. Sideways Lunge Adductor Stretch

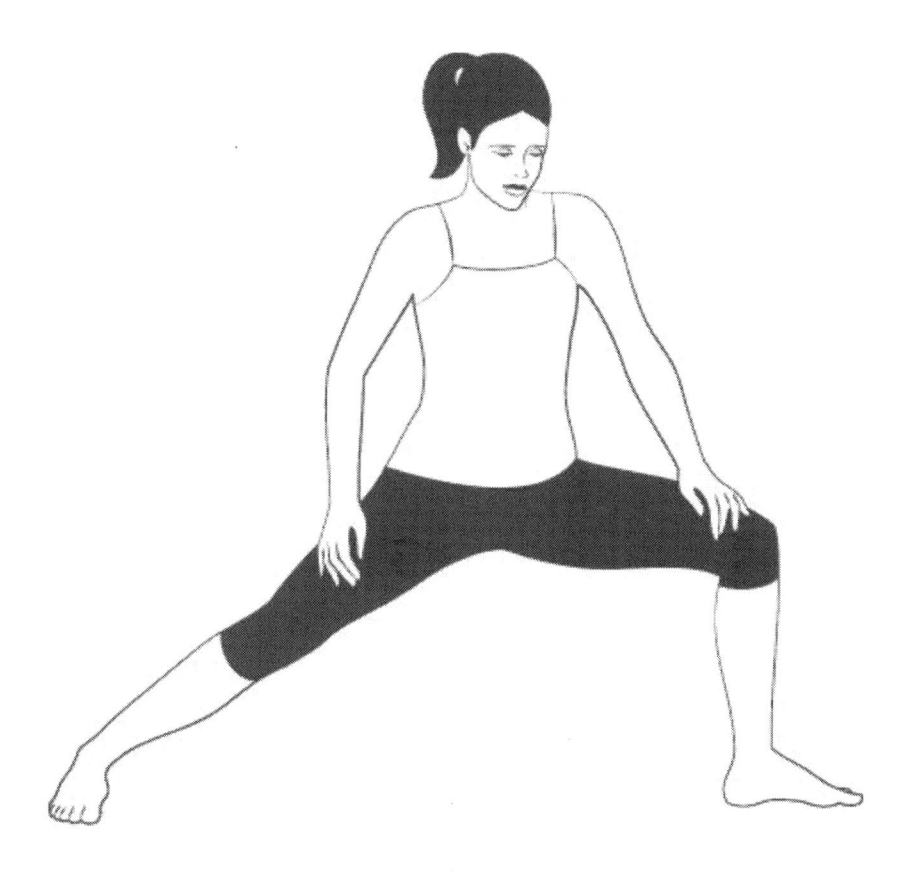

To perform the sideways lunge, keep the rear foot sideways and flat on the floor, and bend the front leg gently, until you feel a gentle stretch along the inside of your leg.

Keep your body upright—there is no need to lean forward. Hold this stretch for 30 seconds, and then repeat with your other leg.

7. Hip Flexor Stretch

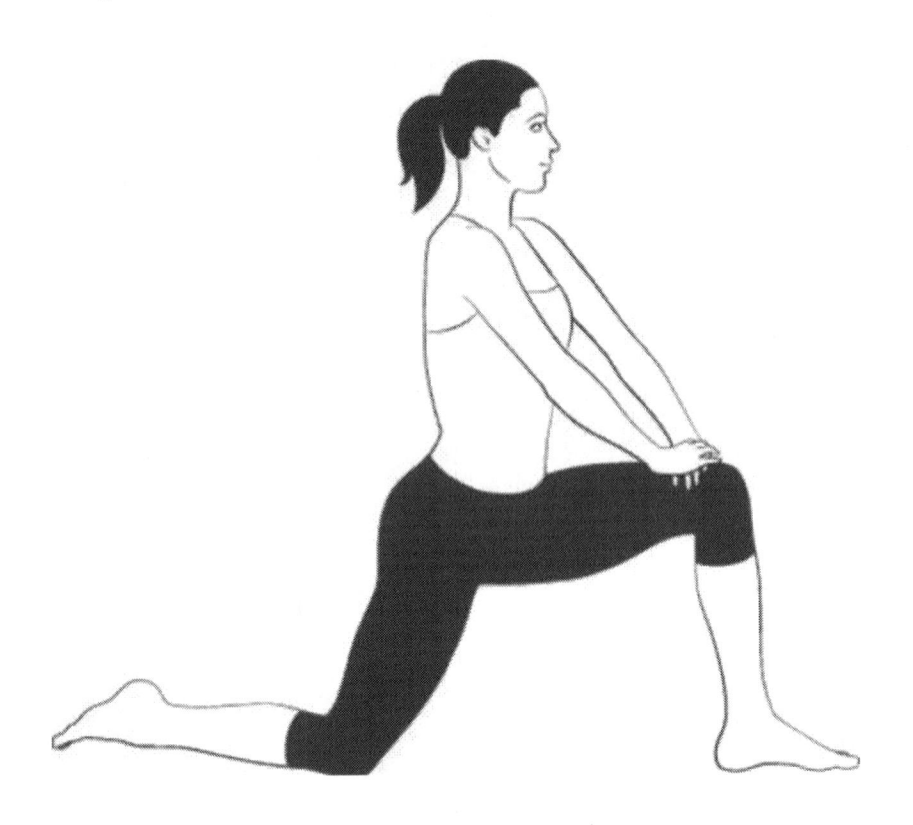

First kneel onto your right knee, with toes down, and place your left foot flat on the floor in front of you.

Place both hands on your left thigh and press your hips forward until you feel a good stretch in the hip flexors.

Contract your abdominals and slightly tilt your pelvis back while keeping your chin parallel to the floor. Hold this pose for 20 to 30 seconds, and then switch sides.

You'll probably remember that the hip flexor stretch is also good for reversing bad posture (see Way #3)!

8a. Quadriceps Lying Down Stretch

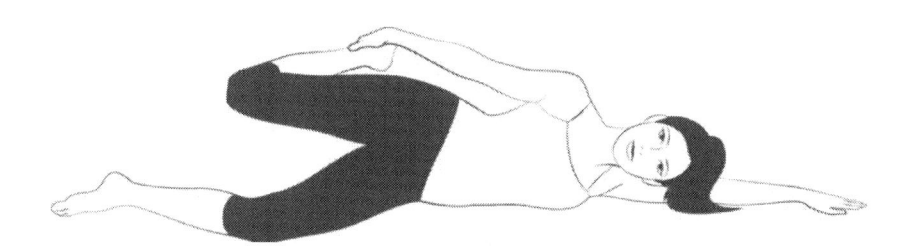

Lie on your side and contract your abdominals, before grasping the top of your foot and bringing it toward your glutes. Hold this stretch for 30 seconds, and then repeat with your other leg.

8b. Quadriceps Stretch (Contract-Relax Version)

Bring your ankle toward your glutes. For 7 to 10 seconds, attempt to straighten your leg, but let your hands "win."

Relax and then stretch the ankle back toward the glutes for 7 to 10 seconds. Repeat this stretch two to three times.

9. Total Back Stretch

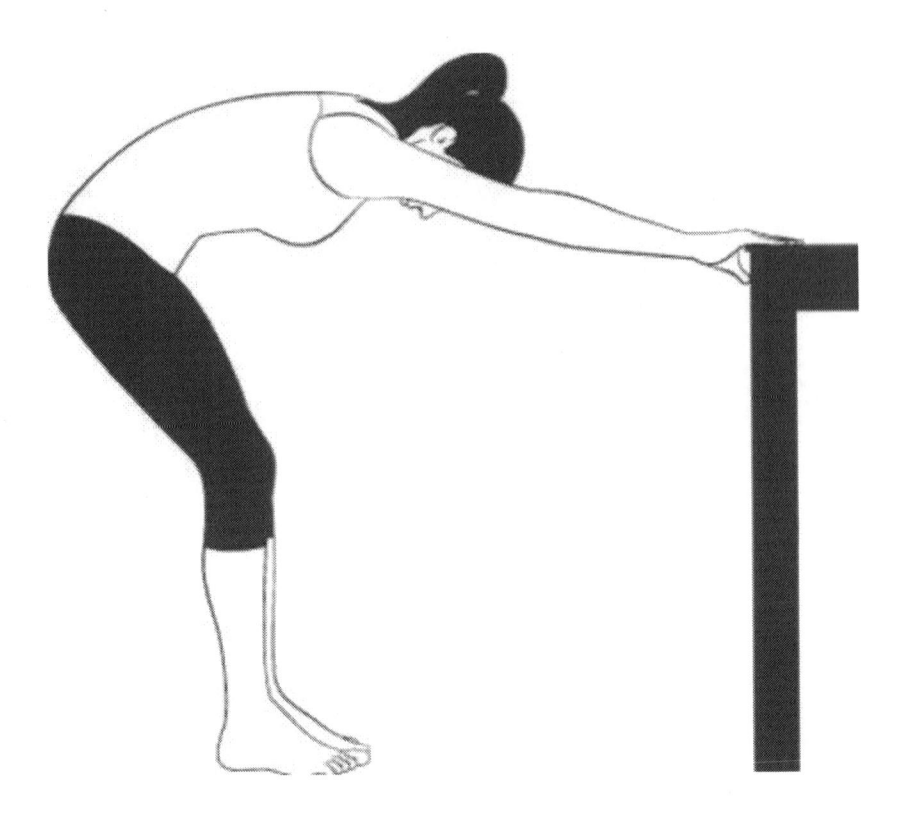

Stand a few feet away from a doorknob or handrail on a stairwell. Grasp the edge and pull while curling forward and stretching the back muscles.

SUCCESS! You should be experiencing noticeable low back pain relief.

Way #6: Pose like a Yogi

Practicing the following yoga poses can help lengthen your spine, stretch and strengthen your muscles and return your back to its proper alignment.

Seven Back-Saving Yoga Poses

1. Downward-Facing Dog

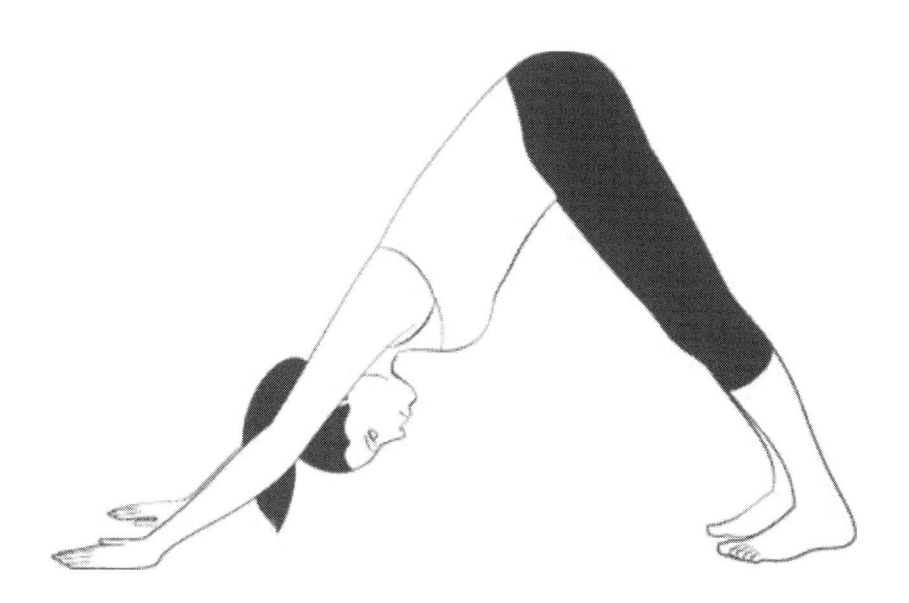

Start on your hands and knees, with your hands slightly in front of your shoulders.

Pressing back, raise your knees away from the floor and lift your tailbone up toward the ceiling. For an added hamstring stretch, gently push your heels toward the floor.

Hold the position for five to ten breaths, and then repeat the pose five to seven times.

DIY Low Back Pain Relief

What's It Good For?

Besides stretching the hamstrings and calves, the Downward-Facing Dog pose increases flexibility in the upper back and shoulders, while at the same time building upper-body strength.

2. Upward Dog

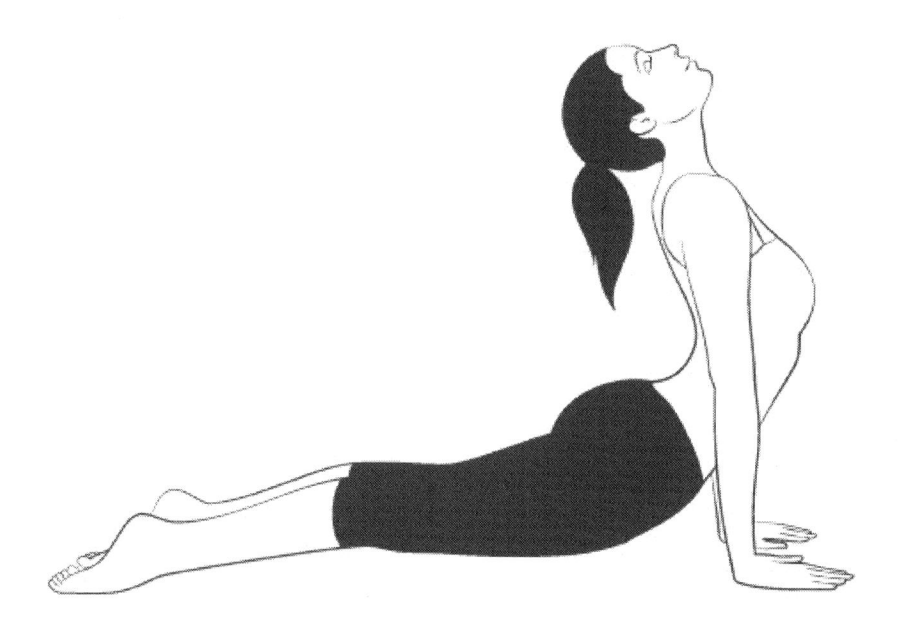

To start, lie face down with your legs straight out. Bend your arms and rest your palms on the floor on either side of your chest. Look straight ahead of you.

Take a deep breath in and shrug your shoulders up to your ears. Squeeze your shoulder blades together.

Now exhale and press your hands down and straighten your arms. Bring your torso and legs off the floor, evenly distributing your weight between your hands and toes.

Try to elongate your body, while keeping your neck long.

Hold the Upward Dog pose for several breaths and repeat the pose five to seven times.

What's It Good For?

Upward Dog improves the posture by stretching the chest, shoulders and reversing the desk jockey's notorious anterior pelvic tilt. It also strengthens the spine, arms and wrists. Another great benefit is that it tightens the glutes, which often get weak from a sedentary lifestyle.

3. Child's Pose

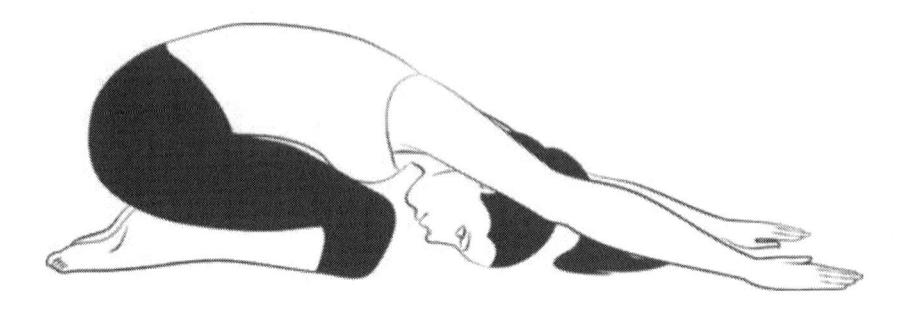

Start on all fours with your arms stretched out straight in front of you, then sit back so your glutes come to rest just above—but not touching—your heels.

Hold the position for five to ten breaths.

What's It Good For?

Child's Pose helps to lengthen and stretch the spine, while relieving neck and low back pain. It also gently stretches the hips, thighs, ankles and the muscles, tendons and ligaments in the knee.

4. Pigeon Pose

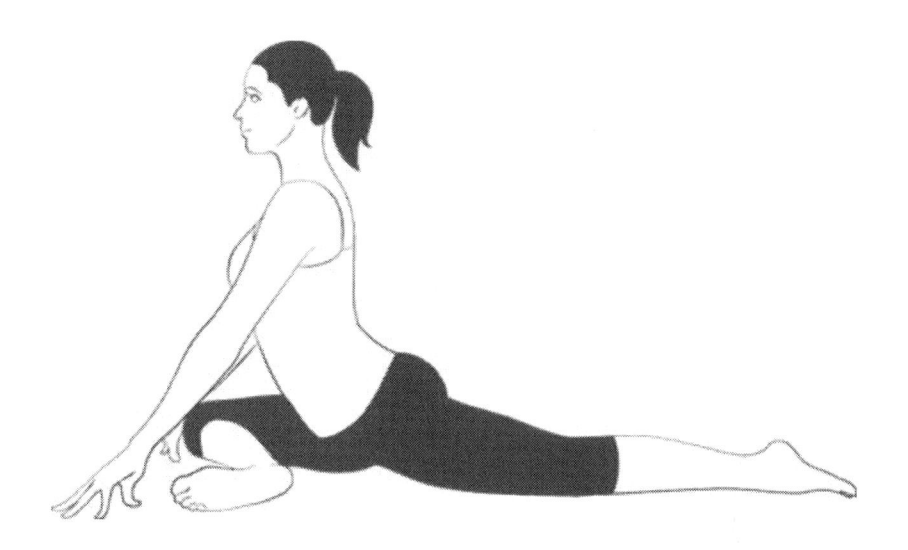

Start in Downward-Facing Dog pose with your feet together.

Draw your right knee forward and turn it out to the right, so your right leg is bent and your left leg is extended straight behind you.

Slowly lower both legs.

Hold the position for five to ten breaths, and then switch to the other side.

What's It Good For?

Pigeon Pose can stretch deep into the glutes, releasing the tension in the piriformis, which, as mentioned earlier, can cause sciatic pain. The groin (adductors) and psoas muscles also get a healthy stretch with the Pigeon Pose.

5. Triangle Pose

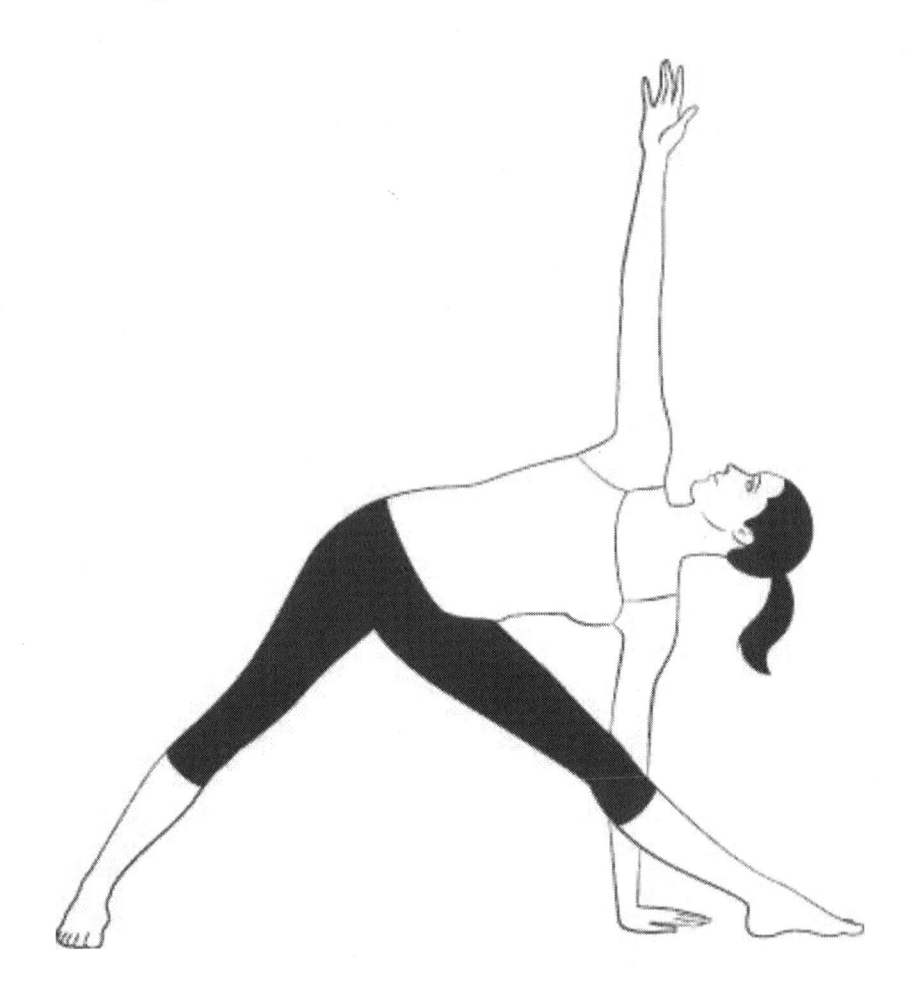

Start standing straight with your feet together.

Lunge your right foot back 3 to 4 feet, and pivot and point your right foot out at a 45-degree angle.

Turn your chest to the right side and open the pose by stretching your left arm toward the floor and the right arm toward the ceiling, keeping both your right and left legs straight. You might not be able to touch the floor with your

Way #6: Pose like a Yogi

right arm at first, so don't overstretch—only bend as far as you can while maintaining a straight back.

Hold the position for five to ten breaths, and then switch to the other side.

What's It Good For?

Triangle Pose helps to both stretch and strengthen a plethora of muscles, including the legs, knees, ankle joints, hips, groin muscles, hamstrings, calves, shoulders, chest and spine.

6. Cat & Cow Poses

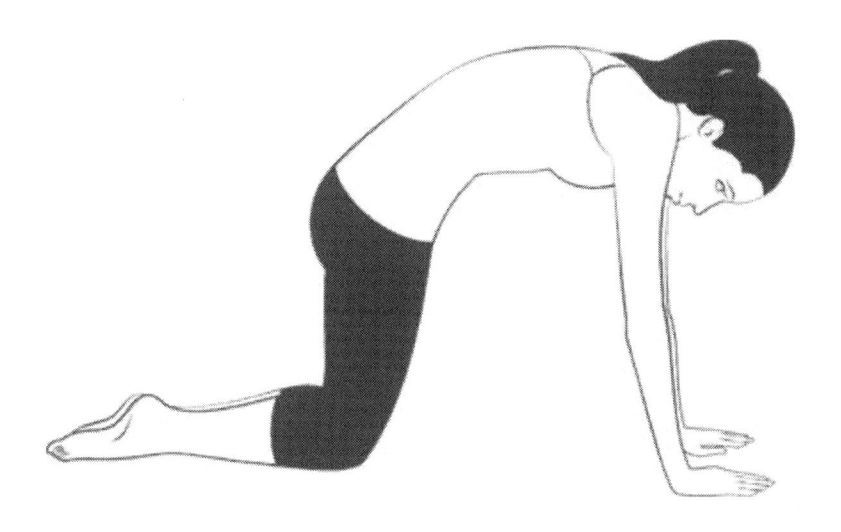

Starting on your hands and knees, an all-fours position, move into the Cat Pose by slowly pressing your spine up, arching your back.

Hold the pose for a few seconds, and then move to the Cow Pose by scooping your spine in, pressing your shoulder blades back and lifting your head.

Moving back and forth from Cat Pose to Cow Pose helps move your spine to a neutral position, relaxing the muscles and easing tension.

Repeat the sequence 10 times, flowing smoothly from cat to cow, and cow back to cat.

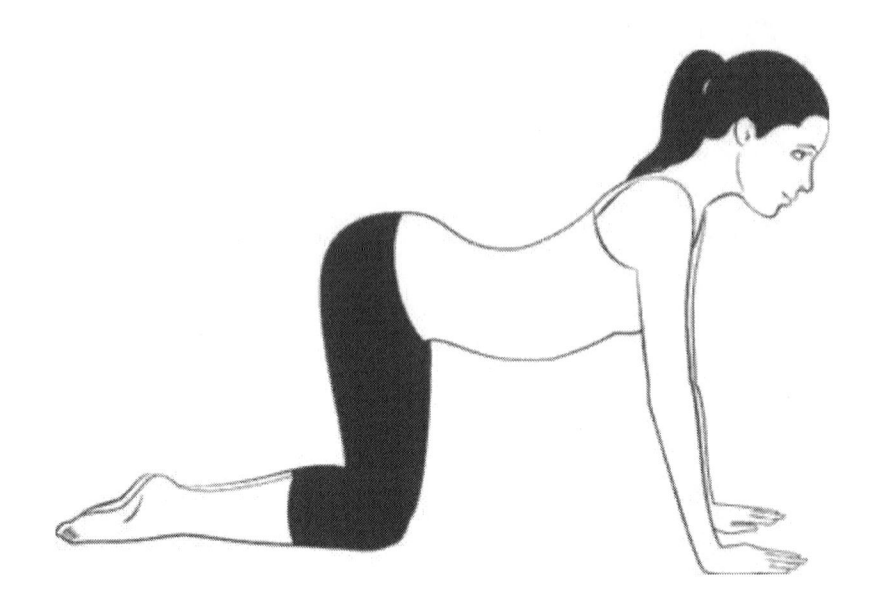

What's It Good For?

Cat and Cow Poses are great for improving posture and balance. It stretches the hips, abdomen, neck and back, while simultaneously strengthening the spine and neck.

7. Cobra Pose

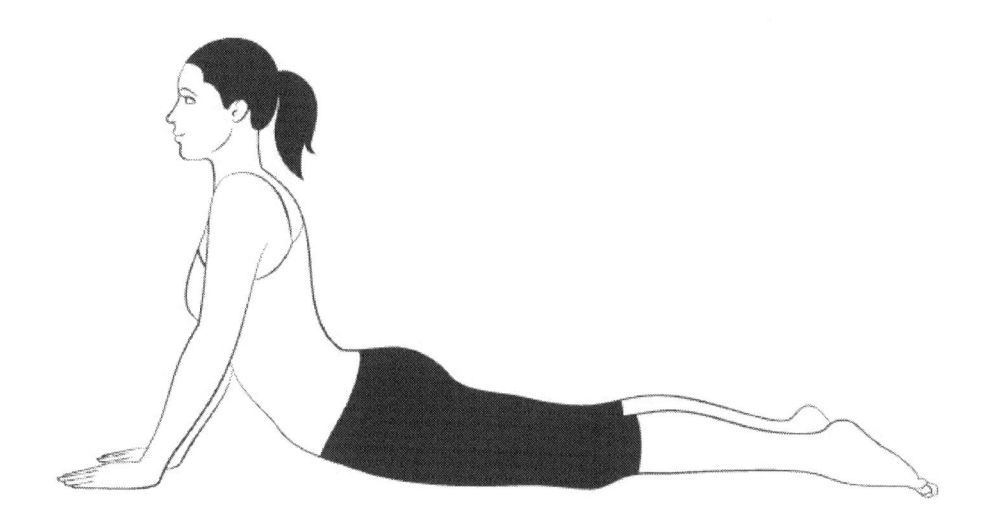

Start by lying flat on the floor with your palms face down near the middle of your ribs.

While drawing your legs together and pressing the tops of your feet into the floor, use the strength of your back, not your hands, to lift your chest off the floor.

Leave your legs extended straight at first.

Hold the position for five to ten breaths.

What's It Good For?

Similar to Upward Dog, the Cobra Pose reduces neck and back pain by stretching and opening up chronically tight muscles, such as the shoulders, chest and neck. This pose also stretches the abdominals and reduces the chances of sciatica by increasing flexibility in your lower back, hips and legs.

Namaste.

Way #7: Roll Out the Knots on Your Own

Stretching is not enough when it comes down to releasing a knotted muscle. If you can't carve out the time to schedule a professional, deep tissue massage, or you can't fit one into your budget, performing a self-massage with a tennis ball or foam roller can be a cost-effective alternative.

Self-Massage Technique #1: The Tennis-Ball Method

Using a tennis ball (or lacrosse ball) to work out the knots and tight spots in the low back is a time-honored pastime for many self-massage enthusiasts. Tennis balls can easily grip the skin and sink in and loosen up the thoraco-lumbar fascia (that's the connective tissue in the low back).

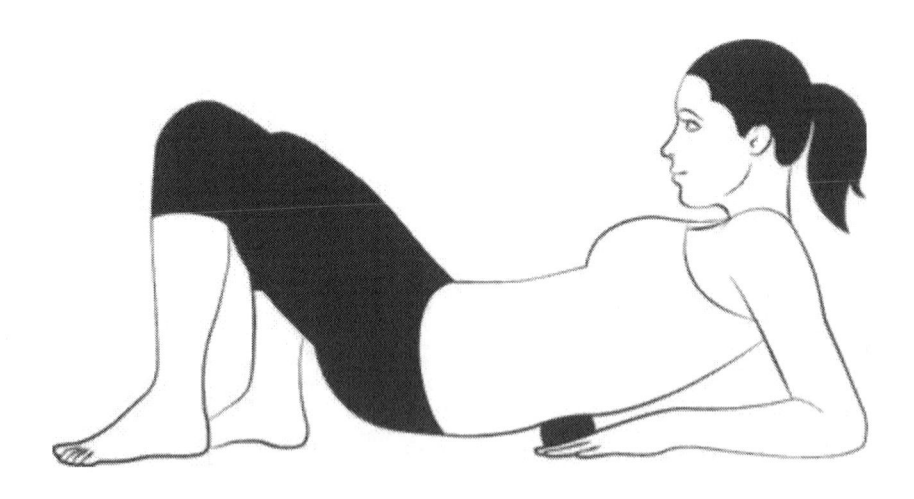

Start by lying on the floor and propping yourself up on your elbows. Then lift up your bottom and place two tennis balls on either side of your lower spine.

Let your body slowly ease onto the two balls, and then use your arms to help you glide down toward your heels and then

Way #7: Roll Out the Knots on Your Own

back up just below your ribcage and then back down again. Continue doing this for 90 seconds, or about 8 to 12 repetitions.

If this position starts to strain your neck and shoulders, rest your head and upper body on the floor and place the balls in the groove on either side of your lower spine. Then rock your hips side to side, like an excited dog slowly wagging its tail. You should feel the tension and tightness in your low back melt away.

Got a Pain in the Butt? Try This!

You can try self trigger-point therapy using a ball. Find a painful spot in the glutes, place the ball at that location and then relax your body into the ball.

Hold this position for 30 to 60 seconds or until you notice a significant reduction in pain. Move to the next painful spot. The total time spent on this exercise should be between 5 and 10 minutes.

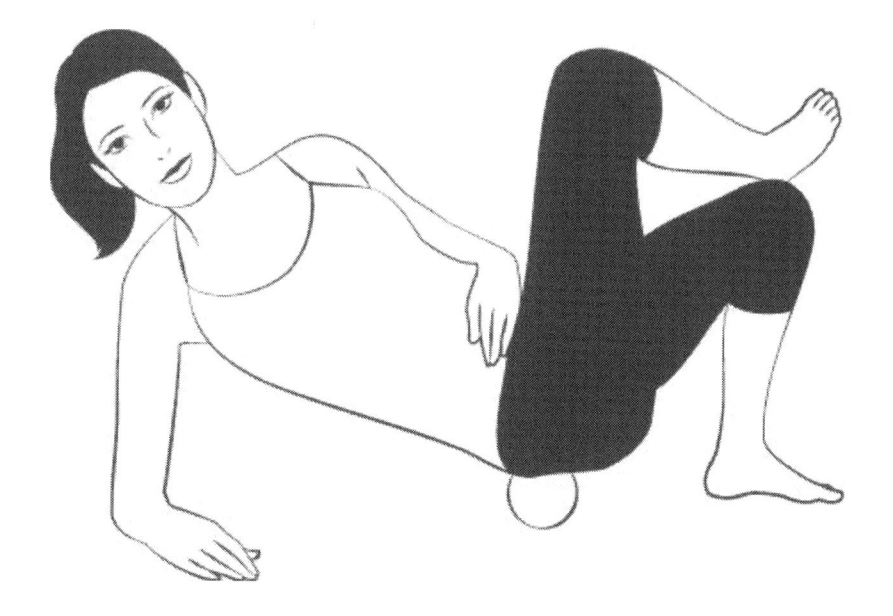

That's how you roll your low back pain away. And then, of course, book a massage to make sure all the knots have been annihilated.

Self-Massage Technique #2: The Foam-Roller Method

Myofascial foam rolling can help break down adhesions and scar tissue in the soft tissues of the muscles. Using the weight of your own body, the cylindrical foam roller[5] can provide a myofascial release self-massage, smoothing the trigger points, while increasing blood flow and circulation to the soft tissues.

Researchers at Memorial University in Canada published a paper in the January 2014 edition of Medicine & Science in Sports & Exercise on the effects of foam rolling as a recovery tool after intense physical activity. The researchers found that foam rolling was beneficial at improving range of motion and reducing delayed onset muscle soreness felt immediately after a hard workout.

When using a foam roller, search for tender areas or trigger points and roll onto these areas, controlling the intensity with your own body weight. Depending on the muscle that you're targeting, you might have to position the roller in a parallel or perpendicular direction, or at a 45-degree angle.

---

[5] You can purchase this item at a fitness center, athletic store, department store, or online.

Way #7: Roll Out the Knots on Your Own

Seven Foam-Roller Moves to Conquer Back Pain

1. Low Back (part 1)

Start out by placing the foam roller underneath your low back. Maintain a neutral spine by tucking your abs and placing your hands behind your knees. Slowly roll up and down the foam roller 10 to 12 times.

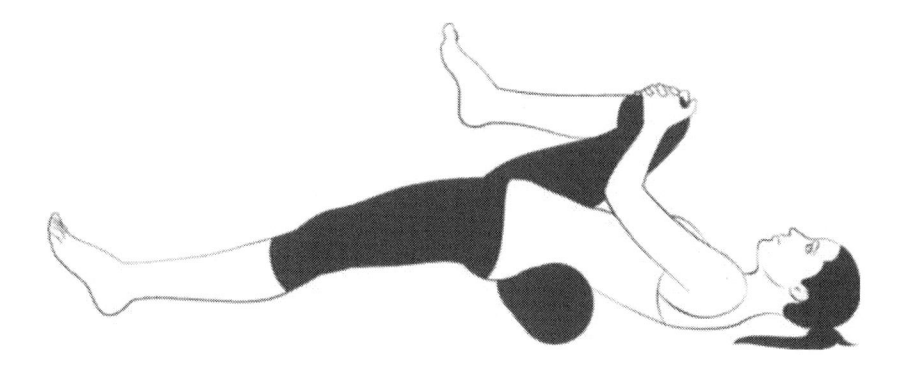

2. Low Back (part 2)

With the foam roller resting underneath your low back, pull your right leg up and hug your right knee. Roll from the base of your left side of your rib cage to above your glutes. Do 10 to 12 slow and steady passes, and then repeat on the other side.

3. Hamstrings

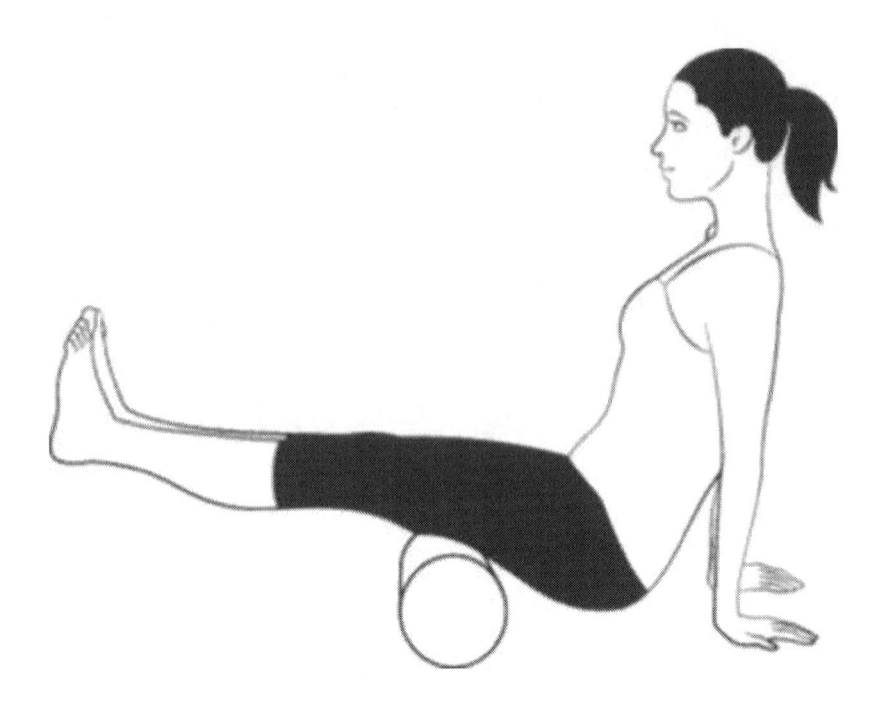

Place the foam roller underneath your upper hamstring muscles below your glutes. Cross your right leg over your left leg and roll the foam roller from your glutes down to right above your left knee. Do 10 to 12 slow and steady passes. Repeat on the other side.

4. Glutes

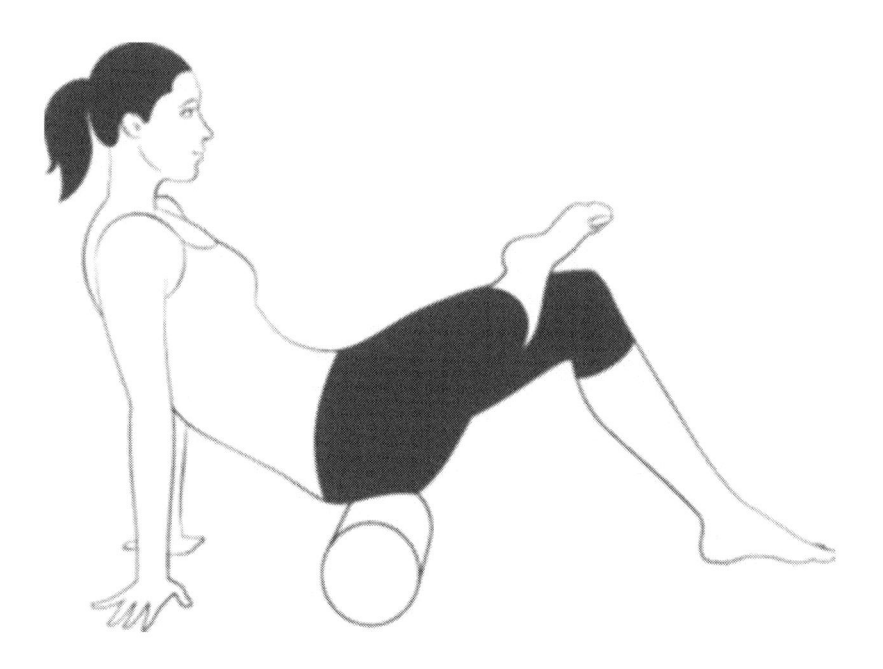

With the foam roller resting underneath both your glutes, bring your right leg up and rest your right ankle above your left knee. Roll onto the side of your right hip. Do 10 to 12 slow and steady passes. Repeat on the other side.

5. The IT Band

The IT band (iliotibial band) is a thick, strong band of fascia that spans from the top of the hipbone down the thighbone to the side of the knee. If a person has tight glutes, this can pull the IT band back and alter the pelvic tilt and cause muscle imbalances.

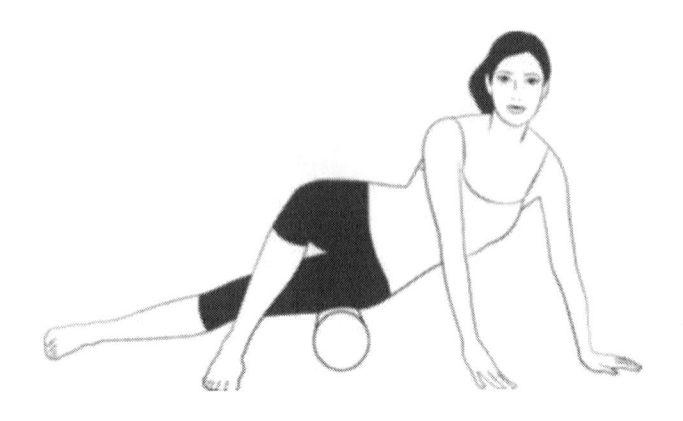

Start by lying on your side with the foam roller underneath the upper thigh. With the assistance of your legs and arms, roll the length of your IT band along the foam roller from the outside, upper portion of your thigh to just above your knee. Do 10 to 12 passes. Repeat on the other side.

Way #7: Roll Out the Knots on Your Own

6. Quadriceps and Hip Flexors

Because your hip flexors are located slightly toward the outer portion of your pelvic region, it's more effective to roll with just one thigh rather than on both sides at the same time.

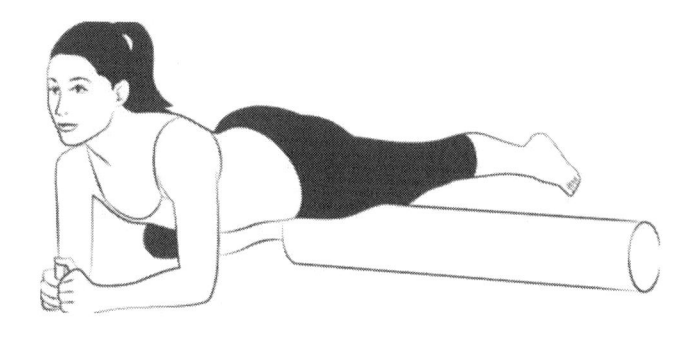

Start facedown on the floor in a plank position with one thigh on the foam roller. As you roll up and down on your hip flexors, slightly rotate right to left to seek and destroy any knots or trigger points. Continue until you hit the entire front side of your thigh. Do 10 to 12 slow and steady passes up and down the quad. Repeat on the other side.

7. Adductors

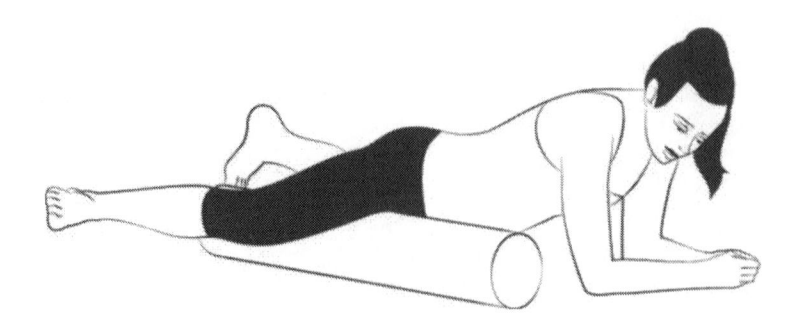

Roll the foam roller along the inner thigh region as high as you're comfortable. Find the tightest spot and lie on it for about 30 to 60 seconds.

Phew! I bet you're happy that's over. Remember, you're in control, and if the pain is too much to handle, back off and work on that area another time.

Way #8: Sleep This Way

A 2011 study evaluating pain and sleep, published in *European Spine Journal*, found that 58.7 percent of people suffering with low back pain experienced sleep disturbance. I've had countless clients who come to me saying that they woke up feeling stiff and achy, probably from "sleeping wrong."

What IS the Right Way to Sleep if You Have Low Back Pain?

Lying on your side with a pillow between your knees will help to reduce any curve in your spine and ease the pressure on your spinal discs.

Check Your Bed

According to a 2010 study in *Applied Ergonomics*, if you have low back pain, getting a medium to firm mattress layered with memory foam might be the best choice for reducing your pain and improving your quality of sleep.

If your current mattress is more than 10 years old, it's probably time to get a new one. An old, lumpy bed and the position you sleep in can cause your back to become strained during that valuable rest-time. This "can actually increase stress on our ligaments, spinal discs and spinal joints," says Dr. Robert Oexman, director of the Sleep to Live Institute.[6]

---

[6] This quote and those in the following paragraph are from http://www.huffingtonpost.com/2012/05/08/back-pain-bed-stretches_n_1452898.html

DIY Low Back Pain Relief

Before You Roll Out of Bed . . .

When your alarm clock rings or buzzes in the morning, do you leap out of bed like you've been struck by lightning, or do you hit the snooze button?

Dr. Oexman says your answer should be, "Stretch my back!" He says that the "greatest incidence of slipped discs occurs within 30 to 60 minutes after we wake up."

Oexman recommends that you "stretch out your back before you ever leave bed" instead of falling back to sleep, which interrupts your natural sleep pattern, counteracting sleep's restorative values.

The following four stretches can make a powerful difference in preventing back pain and keeping you limber throughout the day.

Way #8: Sleep This Way

Don't Roll Out of Bed before You Do These Four Stretches

1. Low Back

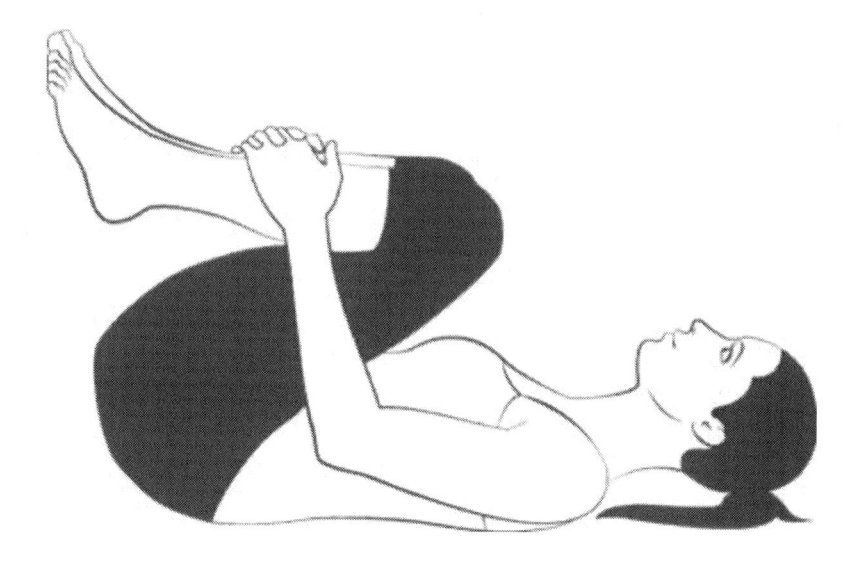

Bring both your knees to your chest. Start by first raising one and then holding the knee with both hands. Then raise the other knee. Grasping both your knees, pull them toward your chest. Hold each stretch for 2 seconds and repeat 10 times.

2. Piriformis Stretch

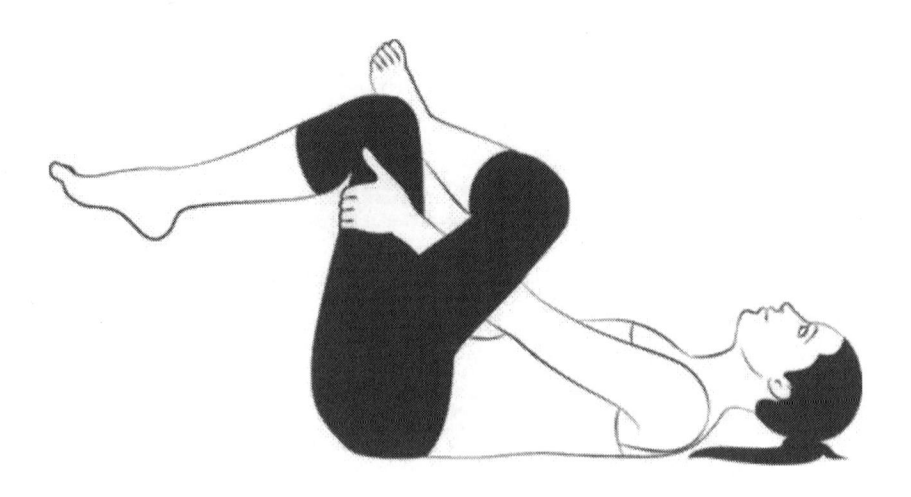

The piriformis muscle runs through the glutes and can contribute to back and leg pain.

Lying on your back with both knees bent, cross your left leg over your right leg. Using both hands, reach under your right knee and pull it toward your chest. You should feel a stretch in the glutes on your left side. Repeat on the opposite side.

There are two methods of holding this stretch. One is the active-isolated version, where you hold each stretch for 2 seconds and repeat 10 times. The other method involves holding a static stretch for 30 seconds and repeating it three times. Try both methods and choose which works best for you.

3. Pelvic Tilt

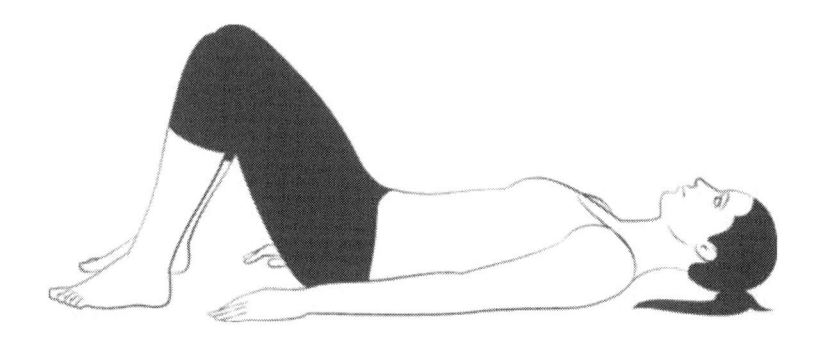

Lie on your back with your knees bent. In this relaxed position, the small of your back will not be touching the floor. Tighten your abdominal muscles so that the small of your back presses against the floor. Hold this pose for 5 seconds, and then relax. Repeat this three times and gradually build to 10 repetitions. You'll remember this from Way #5 to help stretch your back!

4. Knees to Chest

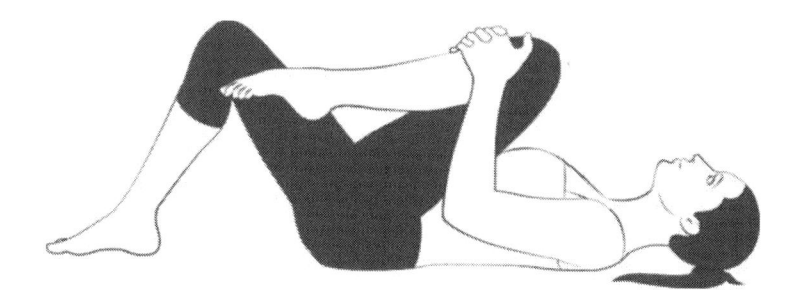

Lie on your back with both legs straight out. Bring one knee to your chest and do a pelvic tilt. Hold for 2 seconds and repeat 10 times. Repeat with the opposite leg.

Now, you can confidently roll out of bed the right way.

Way #9a: Get a Deep Tissue Massage

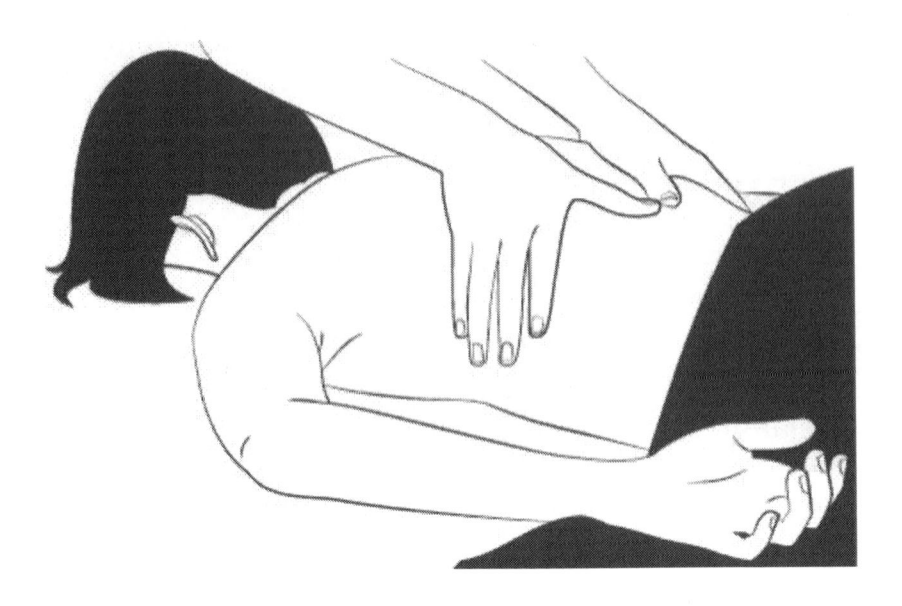

Evidence suggests that massage is one of the most promising drug-free and surgery-free methods for treating low back pain.

The Evidence

According to a 2011 low back pain study published in the Annals of Internal Medicine, researchers at the Group Health Research Institute found that getting a Swedish or structural massage was beneficial to help alleviate chronic low back pain.

After receiving one massage a week for 10 weeks, one out of three patients with chronic low back pain improved and were pain free, compared to one out of twenty-five patients who were given the "usual care." Usual care applies to any doctor-recommended treatment, including painkillers, anti-inflammatory drugs, muscle relaxants, or physical therapy.

Way #9a: Get a Deep Tissue Massage

The massage ultimately helped the study participants with low back pain even after six months, allowing them to remain active and productive.

"This is important because chronic back pain is among the most common reasons people see doctors and alternative practitioners, including massage therapists," says Dr. Daniel Cherkin, a senior investigator at Group Health Research Institute. "It's also a common cause of disability, absenteeism, and 'presenteeism,' when people are at work but can't perform well."[7]

Deep Tissue Massage Is Statistically Better for Low Back Pain Relief than Therapeutic Massage

A small Polish study featuring 26 patients indicated that deep tissue massage is "statistically" more beneficial at treating low back pain as compared with therapeutic massage, although "further research is needed to verify the results," the researchers noted in their 2012 *Studies in Health Technology and Informatics* article.

This study compared the effectiveness of two different massage modalities on chronic low back pain—the gentler, Swedish-style therapeutic massage and, my personal favorite, deep tissue massage. The research was conducted on 26 patients, from age 60 to 75 years, who were separated into two groups. The study participants received massage for 10 days, for 30-minute sessions each day.

The results showed that participants with low back pain who received deep tissue massage experienced significantly more relief than the group who received therapeutic massage.

---

[7] See http://www.grouphealthresearch.org/news-and-events/newsrel/2011/110704.html

So How Does Deep Tissue Massage Break Up the Chronic Pain Cycle?

Breaking chronic pain's vicious cycle of pain and muscle spasm is not an easy task. The cycle goes like this: pain causes muscle tension, which leads to decreased circulation and range of motion, all of which increase the pain. This brings about even more tension, and even less circulation, inducing more pain, securing the cycle.

The body's natural reaction to any contracted area with poor circulation is to lay down connective tissue (also known as collagen fibers, the building blocks of scar tissue). Despite the healing nature of this process, the body inevitably "glues" the muscles and their connective tissue coverings into a shortened state. This tightness can leave you feeling stiff, restricted, tired and sore.

These tight muscles can often develop trigger points, which are hyperirritable spots that refer pain and tingling to other places in the body. These trigger points can press on nerves, causing numbness and tingling, and even more pain.

Using a deeper pressure than the standard therapeutic massage, deep tissue massage helps to release the cranky trigger points and break up the muscle adhesions. In my practice, I use a pain scale with my clients to assess the level of pressure I'm applying. I watch and listen to the client as I massage them, and promptly lighten up if I sense the pressure is too much, or if they verbally tell me.

Can Deep Tissue Massage Help with Herniated Discs?

Massage therapy isn't a magic pill and can't reverse the curse of a current disc herniation. However, massage CAN be extremely helpful in reducing pain by loosening the tight low back muscles that compress and pinch the underlying discs.

Way #9a: Get a Deep Tissue Massage

As with any potentially serious medical condition, I always recommend getting approval from a doctor before booking a massage.

Massage Can Reduce Low Back Pain, So Falling Asleep Can Be as Easy as 1-2-Zzzzz!

There's no doubt that massage helps you relax, but did you know that it can improve your sleep? Numerous studies have delved into this connection and credit it to massage's effect on delta waves, the kind of brain waves connected to deep sleep, according to *Health Magazine*.

A 2007 randomized study by the Touch Research Institute evaluated the effects of massage therapy versus relaxation therapy on chronic low back pain. Treatment effects were evaluated for reducing pain, depression, anxiety and sleep disturbances, for improving trunk range of motion and for reducing job absenteeism and increasing job productivity.

After a 30-minute massage twice a week for five weeks, the study participants in the massage therapy group reported experiencing less pain, depression, anxiety, sleep disturbance and improved range of motion.

In summary, getting a massage at least twice a week can yield positive results for low back pain sufferers and improve their overall quality of life.

How Has Deep Tissue Massage Helped My Clients with Back Pain?

Here's what some of my massage clients suffering chronic low back pain have said about how my deep tissue massages have helped them:

I have been going to Morgan Massage since 2005 and would not even consider another massage therapist. Within a couple of months of going to him back in 2005, the upper back pain I had suffered from for so many years (from computer work) was basically eliminated, just from regular deep tissue massages. Prior to seeing Morgan, I had been to numerous doctors, physical therapists, and acupuncturists for the same problem. Deep tissue massage was the answer—I wish I had known about Morgan earlier.

—Anne B.

Morgan did a fabulous job of dealing with my acute back pain. After just a few sessions, my pain is almost entirely gone. I am looking forward to getting back to 100%, but the improvement has been phenomenal already.

—Tom M.

I have seen Morgan for over two years. The last time I came in, I had thrown out my back. I have had two herniated discs. He really helped relieve pain and loosen up my joints. Cannot say enough good things. Superb.

—Drew L.

I came to Morgan Massage with a lot of stiffness in my lower back and legs due to the herniation in my lower back. After the first massage I started feeling much looser in my achy muscles and got some back pain relief and hoping for more in the future sessions. Morgan is very attentive to your body needs. I have never had better messages and would definitely recommend it.

—Ana S.

This visit to Morgan was to relieve sciatic nerve pain shooting down my right leg. In addition to his usual focused massage techniques, this time he introduced specific stretches and

Way #9a: Get a Deep Tissue Massage

cupping as an integral part of the session. I'm not 100% yet but I'm certainly on my way, thanks to Morgan's deep understanding of muscle interaction and anatomy.

—Ethan W.

Way #9b: Enhance Your Massage with Cupping

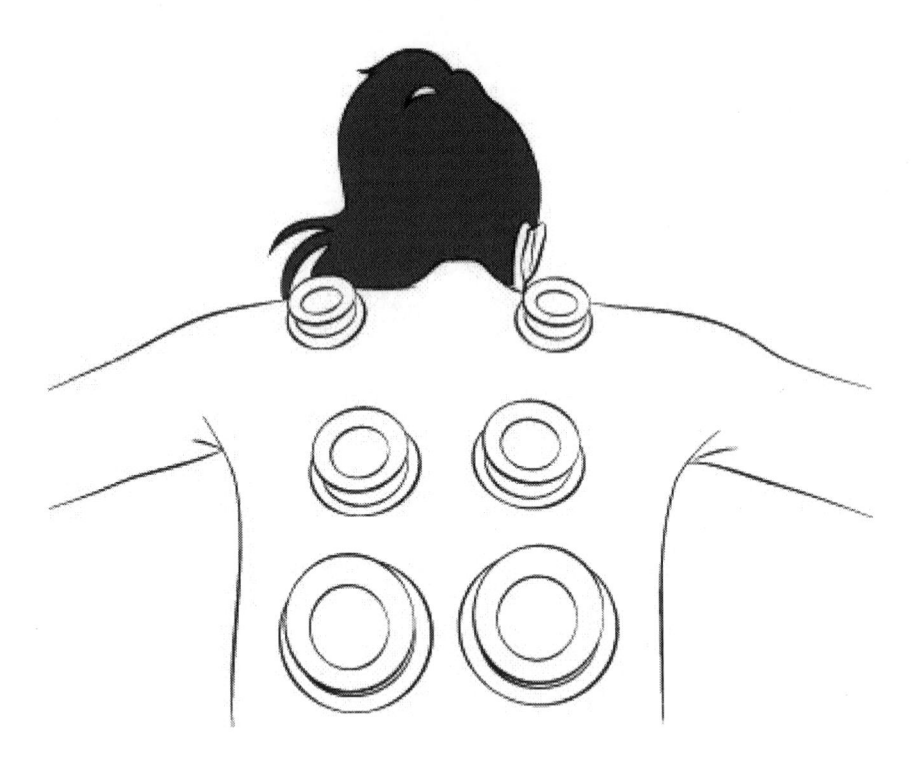

The strong suction of massage cupping with silicone cups is similar to the skin rolling of a deep tissue massage, but without the pain. When treating clients who suffer from low back pain, the silicone cups allow me to go deep without causing my clients pain.

The silicone cups literally become an extension of my hands, allowing me to decompress and create negative pressure, which seamlessly lifts and loosens restricted muscle adhesions versus performing the classic compression of massage.

Way #9b: Enhance Your Massage with Cupping

I'm able to achieve immediate results, bringing a pain scale of 9 to a 1 or 2 in a matter of minutes. Achieving these profound therapeutic results is simply not possible with hands alone. It's said that 5 minutes of cupping is equivalent to 30 minutes of a deep tissue massage.

Cupping along the spine stimulates the parasympathetic nervous system, producing a relaxing and sedating effect on the recipient and it's not uncommon for them to fall asleep. Toxic feelings of anxiety and stress are literally lifted up and away.

Traditionally performed in a Chinese medicine setting to enhance acupuncture treatments, cupping methods have evolved with the therapeutic application and modernization of the equipment. The original use of hollowed out animal horns (the Horn Method) was used to treat boils and suck out toxins of snakebites and skin lesions. The horns slowly evolved to bamboo cups, which were eventually replaced by glass, then plastic and now silicone cups.

Cupping has been around for thousands of years. In fact, 2,500 years ago, Hippocrates, the father of modern medicine, raved about cupping and how it was a cure-all for every disease. Even Hippocrates' contemporaries were known to use the strong suction of cupping to restore spinal alignments by reducing dislocated vertebrae from protruding inward.

A Hot New Celebrity Trend

In 2004, at a New York film festival, the limelight was on actress Gwyneth Paltrow's back, revealing fresh cupping marks. Countless celebrities, such as Jennifer Aniston, Victoria Beckham, Denise Richards, Hilary Rhoda, and Nicole Richie followed suit and became fast adopters of this hot new cupping trend. Unfortunately, some of the Hollywood buzz viewed the celeb's cupping marks as simply bruises and rolled their eyes at its potential benefits.

Until recently, there was scant published evidence in favor of cupping for pain relief. During the past three years, however, a handful of new studies have shown it helps relieve back, neck, carpal tunnel and knee pain.

In one 40-person study of neck pain caused by computer use, "cupping therapy was effective in reducing pain," says Tae-Hun Kim, a researcher at the Korea Institute of Oriental Medicine in Daejeon, South Korea.[8] The study, published online in the *Journal of Occupational Health*, found that six cupping sessions over two weeks was more effective on average in relieving pain than a heating pad—and the benefit lasted a month after treatment ended.

What about Those Cupping Marks?

Cupping can leave marks, which simply means that the stagnation has been moved from the deeper tissue layers to the superficial layers, allowing fresh oxygenated blood to nourish and heal the underlying tissues. When a cup is left long enough in one place, not only will it loosen up any muscular tension, but it will also pull up to the skin surface any local build-up of waste products, such as stagnant blood, lymph and toxins.

Cupping marks are commonly mistaken as bruises, but that just isn't the case. Bruising is caused by impact trauma with the breakage of capillaries and a reactionary rush of fluids to the damaged location from the tissue injury. With properly performed cupping, there's no compression involved, only decompression.

---

[8] See http://online.wsj.com/news/articles/SB10001424127887324073504578114970824081566

Way #9b: Enhance Your Massage with Cupping

How Long Do The Marks Last?

The marks can range in color from a bright red to dark purple, usually lasting three days to a week—sometimes longer if the person is extremely sick or sedentary. If there is no stagnation present, there will be only a light pink mark, which disappears in a few minutes to a couple of hours.

Fewer marks will appear as the cupping treatments accumulate. As the stagnation and buildup of unwanted toxins gets released, dispersed and drained, it's less likely to see any discoloration.

While performing massage cupping on my clients with back pain, I've witnessed amazing results, which would be close to impossible by using the human hand alone. One thing is for sure; people who love deep tissue massage will LOVE cupping!

Massage Cupping Testimonials

Chronic Low Back Pain

I've been going to Morgan for about a year and a half every two weeks to help manage the pain from degenerative disc syndrome in my lower back. Additionally, I have been doing cupping work to assist with immune system health. Morgan is a consummate professional who continually seeks to grow his skills and incorporate them into his practice. I would recommend him without question. My back and my immune system are both better thanks to his work.

—Mindy H.

Back Spasm

After vigorous yard work and cleaning out my shed, my lower back was in trouble! I couldn't turn to brush my teeth or lower

DIY Low Back Pain Relief

myself to the sink the next morning . . . I was in spasm. Just 30 minutes of intense massage and cupping I was able to move, turn without pain! It loosened and has been fine since . . . I am so glad Morgan had an opening that day! This has happened before; back, shoulder, headache . . . Morgan is so well trained. He knows exactly what to do the last 15+ years!

—Amy M.

Sciatica Relief

Wow! Wow! Wow! What a great massage. Having gone to several other massage practitioners with limited results I am very satisfied with the results of Morgan's technique. He focused on key areas and you could tell he knew what he was doing. The cupping was a new experience but I like it—and it seemed to loosen up a lot of knots in my back/along my sciatic. I'll be back for sure!"

—Curt S.

Conclusion

Taking ownership of your pain is essential to living a pain-free life and I hope that the nine ways illustrated in this book have empowered you to take action so you can feel like yourself again.

As the old saying goes, "motion is lotion for the joints." What that means is that the older you get, the less lubrication (or synovial fluid) you produce for your joints. And the little fluid you do produce isn't absorbed as well by the joints, so the more active you are, the better you'll feel overall.

Watch some young children, and you'll instantly notice how active they are and how they're naturally inclined to be constantly moving. When recess rolls around, what do they do? Sit on their bums and veg out? Nope! They run around like bolts of lightning and hop, skip and jump.

This is a learning opportunity for back pain sufferers. Instead of resting the back by doing less, activity is essential to reversing the debilitating effects of back pain.

I wish you well on your journey to health and well-being!

References

Introduction

"Handout on Health: Back Pain." (2013). National Institutes of Health (NIH): National Institute of Arthritis and Musculoskeletal and Skin Diseases. See http://www.niams.nih.gov/Health_Info/Back_Pain/default.asp

Hoy, D. Bain, C., Williams, G., March, L., Brooks, P., Blyth, F. Woolf, A., Vos, T., Buchbinder, R. (2012). "A Systemic Review of the Global Prevalence of Low Back Pain." *Arthritis & Rheumatology* 64, no. 6, 2028–2037. doi: 10.1002/art.34347.

Institute of Medicine of the National Academies (2011). *Relieving Pain in America, A Blueprint for Transforming Prevention, Care, Education, and Research.* Washington, DC: The National Academies Press.

"Low Back Pain Fact Sheet." (2003). National Institutes of Health (NIH): National Institute of Neurological Disorders and Stroke. See http://www.ninds.nih.gov/disorders/backpain/detail_backpain.htm.

Malmivaara, A., Häkkinen, U., Aro, T., Heinrichs, M-L., Koskenniemi, L., Kuosma, E., Lappi, S., Paloheimo, R., Servo, C., Vaaranen, V., and Hernberg, S., (1995). "The Treatment of Acute Low Back Pain—Bed Rest, Exercises, or Ordinary Activity?" *The New England Journal of Medicine* 332, 351–355.

References

Way #1: Sit Right

"Low Back Pain Fact Sheet." (2003). National Institutes of Health (NIH): National Institute of Neurological Disorders and Stroke. See http://www.ninds.nih.gov/disorders/backpain/detail_backpain.htm

Way #2: Get Up, Stand Up

Preventing Back Pain at Work and at Home. (2012). American Academy of Orthopaedic Surgeons. See http://orthoinfo.aaos.org/topic.cfm?topic=A00175.

Way #3: Reverse Bad Posture

Lidegaard, M., Jensen, R.B., Andersen, C.H., Zebis, M.K., Colado, J.C. Wang, Y., Heilskov-Hansen, T., and Anderson, L.L. (2013). "Effect of Brief Daily Resistance Training on Occupational Neck/Shoulder Muscle Activity in Office Workers with Chronic Pain: Randomized Controlled Trial." *Biomedical Research International* 262386. doi: 10.115/201/262386.

Way #4: Build a Strong Core

Samartzis, D., Karppinen, J., Chan, D., Luk, K.D.K., and Cheung, K.M.C. (2012). "The Association of Lumbar Intervertebral Disc Degeneration on Magnetic Resonance Imaging with Body Mass Index in Overweight and Obese Adults: A Population-Based Study." *Arthritis & Rheumatology* 64, no. 5, 1488–1496. doi: 10.1002/art.33462.

Shiri, R., Karppinen, J., Leino-Arjas, P., Solovieva, S., and Viikari-Juntura, E. (2010). "The Association between Obesity and Low Back Pain: A Meta-Analysis".

American Journal of Epidemiology 171, no. 2, 135–154. doi: 10.1093/aje/kwp356.

Shiri, R., Solovieva, S., Husgafvel-Pursiainen, K., Taimela, S., Saarikoski, L.A., Huupponen, R., Viikari, J., Raitakari, O.T., and Viikari-Juntura, E. (2008). "The Association between Obesity and the Prevalence of Low Back Pain in Young Adults: The Cardiovascular Risk in Young Finns Study." *American Journal of Epidemiology* 167, no. 9, 1110–1119. doi: 10.1093/aje/kwn007.

Way #7: Roll Out the Knots on Your Own

Macdonald, G.Z., Button, D.C., Drinkwater, E.J., and Behm, D.G. (2014). "Foam Rolling as a Recovery Tool after an Intense Bout of Physical Activity. *Medicine & Science in Sports & Exercise* 46, no. 1, 131–142. doi:10.1249/MSS.0b013e3182a123db.

Way #8: Sleep This Way

Alsaadi, S.M., McAuley, J.H., Hush, J.M., and Maher, C.G. (2011). "Prevalence of Sleep Disturbance in Patients with Low Back Pain. *European Spine Journal* 20, no. 5, 737–743. doi: 10.1007/s00586-010-1661-x.

Jacobson, B.H., Boolani, A., Dunklee, G., Shepardson, A., and Acharya, H. (2010). "Effect of Prescribed Sleep Surfaces on Back Pain and Sleep Quality in Patients Diagnosed with Low Back and Shoulder Pain." *Applied Ergonomics* 42, no. 1, 91–97. doi: 10.1016/j.apergo.2010.05.004.

Way #9a: Get a Deep Tissue Massage

Cherkin, D.C., Sherman, K.J., Kahn, J., Wellman, R., Cook, A.J., Johnson, E., Erro, J., Delaney, K., and Deyo, R.A. (2011). "A Comparison of the Effects of 2 Types of Massage and Usual Care on Chronic Low Back Pain: A Randomized, Controlled Trial." *Annals of Internal Medicine* 155, no. 1, 1–9. doi: 10.7326/0003-4819-155-1-201107050-00002.

References

Field, T., Hernandez-Reif, M., Diego, M., and Fraser, M. (2007). "Lower Back Pain and Sleep Disturbance Are Reduced Following Massage Therapy." *Journal of Bodywork and Movement Therapies* 11, no. 2, 141–145. doi: 10.1016/j.jbmt.2006.03.001.

Lewis, K.K. (2007). "Massage: It's Real Medicine." *Health Magazine.* See http://www.cnn.com/2007/HEALTH/03/08/healthmag.massage/

Romanowski, M., Romanowska, J., and Grześkowiak, M. (2012). "A Comparison of the Effects of Deep Tissue Massage and Therapeutic Massage on Chronic Low Back Pain." *Studies in Health Technology and Informatics* 176, 411–414.

Way #9b: Enhance Your Massage with Cupping

Kim, T.H., Kang, J.W., Kim, K.H., Lee, M.H., Kim, J.E., Kim, J.H., Lee, S., Shin, M.S., Jung, S.Y., Kim, A.R., Park, H.J., and Hong, K.E. (2012). "Cupping for Treating Neck Pain in Video Display Terminal (VDT) Users: A Randomized Controlled Pilot Trial." *Journal of Occupational Health* 54, no. 6, 416–426.

About the Author

Since becoming a professional massage therapist in 2000, Morgan Sutherland has consistently helped thousands of clients manage their back pain with a combination of deep tissue work, cupping and stretching. In 2002, he began a career-long tradition of continuing study by being trained in Tuina—the art of Chinese massage—at the world famous Olympic Training Center in Beijing, China. As an orthopedic massage therapist, Morgan specializes in treating chronic pain and sports injuries and helping restore proper range of motion. In 2006, Morgan became certified as a medical massage practitioner, giving him the knowledge and ability to work with physicians in a complementary healthcare partnership.

When he's not helping clients manage their back pain, he's writing blog posts about pain relief and self care, as well as teaching live and virtual workshops on how to incorporate massage cupping into a bodywork practice. Morgan has received the Angie's List Super Service Award for 2011, 2012, 2013, 2014 and 2015.

Morgan welcomes all comments about your real life experiences implementing the stretches and exercises contained within this book. Thank you for reading ☺

Website: www.morganmassage.com

Email: morgan@morganmassage.com

Facebook page: www.facebook.com/morganmassage